PRINCIPLES AND PRACTICE
OF
PHYSIOLOGIC ACUPUNCTURE

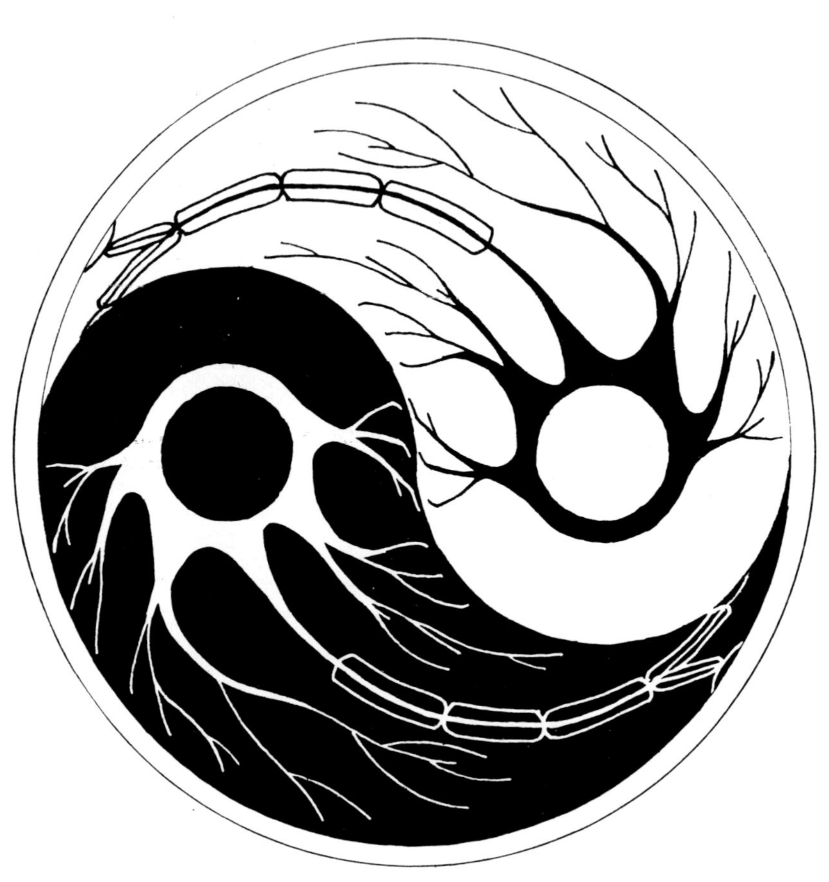

PRINCIPLES AND PRACTICE OF PHYSIOLOGIC ACUPUNCTURE

By

GEORGE A. ULETT, M.D., Ph.D.

Clinical Professor of Psychiatry
St. Louis University School of Medicine

Director
Department of Psychiatry and Neurology
and
Psychosomatic Research Laboratories
Deaconess Hospital
St. Louis, MO

Illustrations by
PACITA CHUA DY, M.D.
and
JUDE McKAY, B.A.

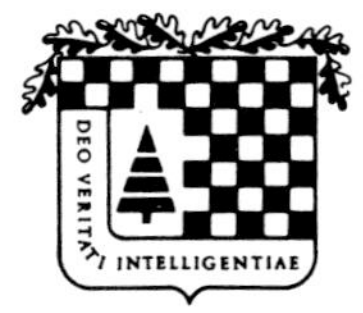

WARREN H. GREEN, INC.
St. Louis, Missouri, U.S.A.

Published by

WARREN H. GREEN, INC.
8356 Olive Blvd.
St. Louis, Missouri 63132, U.S.A.

ISBN No. 0-87527-309-2

Printed in the United States of America

This book is dedicated to Kodo Senshu, M.D., of Tokyo, my first teacher of acupuncture, to Pearl Ulett, M.D., who taught me to appreciate things Chinese and to Tzeng Ze Ming, M.D., who brought acupucture from China to the Phillipines.

Appreciation is expressed to Dr.'s John Stern, Sadishiv Parwatikar, Sven Andersson and Mrs. Margaret Fisher who made suggestions in the original manuscript; to Debra and Esther Schulz for typing the manuscript.

PREFACE

This book has been made possible by recent advances in the neurosciences that permit an explanation of the mechanism of the ancient art of acupuncture in terms concordant with modern medical practice. Clinical experience with acupuncture over many centuries has documented its effectiveness for the relief of pain and other conditions, including some psychosomatic illnesses. Thus it is highly appropriate that acupuncture be presented in such format that it will be more palatable to Western-trained physicians. The theoretical explanations that are the basis of traditional acupuncture have their derivation from the Nei Ching (1,2). That medical manuscript, written between 1000-2000 B.C., is a compilation of all knowledge of acupuncture which had accumulated in the preceding many centuries. Because traditional acupuncture developed at a time when there was no knowledge of physiology and when dissection of the human body was forbidden, it is not surprising that it was explained in metaphysical terms. The diagnosis of disease, selection of sites for needle insertion and the manner of treatment in traditional Chinese medicine were heavily dependent upon numerological and astrological concepts. These theories have been handed down through the years and even today are presented virtually unchanged. Recently published texts on acupuncture still present the techniques and theories in ancient, traditional terminology. Even though some recent texts make mention of possible explanations based on current research findings, they fail to present an acceptable alternate approach for the clinical use of acupuncture. For such reasons, even in the U.S., most who do acupuncture feel that in some mysterious way they are balancing ying and yang, pursuing an evanescent life force, ch'i, through hypothesized (although non-existent) "meridians" and in some cases even making the pretense of palpating the wrist for energy changes produced by distant organ systems of the body. Small wonder then that most scientifically trained physicians have perforce turned their backs on acupuncture.

Some Western physicians have witnessed the production of an acupuncture analgesic effect, sufficient for surgery produced by a few electrically stimulated needles, but have shrugged it off as "hypnosis" or "oriental stoicism." Even when their own patients have experienced relief from chronic pain through acupuncture treatments, many physicians felt it to be "only" placebo response. As a result of continuing publicity in the lay press, increasing numbers of patients with unrelieved chronic pain have sought out and found relief through acupuncture. The demand for acupuncture has thus continued to grow at a rapid pace. This demand has been met primarily by non-medical acupuncturists. Such persons, often deeply steeped in mysticism and lacking sufficient medical knowledge to criticize, have accepted the theories of traditional acupuncture without question. By adhering to those ancient theories they have, thus, applied traditional techniques to the treatment of patients and perpetuated these concepts in their writings and teachings.

It is not surprising that the practice of acupuncture has grown at a fast pace. Patients with unremitting pain and chronic disease are abundant. For many of them Western medicine provides no relief and little hope. Such patients turn readily to esoteric treatments. For reasons to be explained later, traditional acupuncture can give relief to some of these patients. The false and fanciful theories of traditional acupuncture do not impair the effectiveness of needles if they are placed in neuromuscular points and enhanced by electric stimulation. Throughout the history of medicine an empirical treatment has often worked successfully for many years before its mechanism could be explained scientifically. However, when the proper scientific mechanisms were elucidated the treatments could be modified in such a way as to become increasingly effective as, for example, the refinement of drugs to affect specific target organs. Such is the case with acupuncture.

Because of tauted "cure all" claims, traditional unscientific theories and non-medical practitioners, acupuncture was unacceptable to most American physicians. Therefore, state medical licensing boards faced a dilemma in terms of the certification of those who would do acupuncture, often non-physicians. Some boards yielded to pressure and are now in the embarassing position of having established certification procedures for an isolated medical treatment that has been promoted and advertised as a magical remedy for all disease. The examination for such certification is primarily based upon rote memory of the metaphysical concepts of traditional Chinese medicine. Several states permit acupuncture to be practiced only by licensed M.D.'s, D.O.'s, and dentists even though there may be few available who are skilled or even knowledgeable in this treatment methodology. Other states have ignored the matter entirely, perhaps hoping that it was a fad which would soon disappear.

But acupuncture is not a fad. It has survived for some 4,000 years and its success rate in relieving pain is high and incontestable. It has been practiced in Asia for centuries, and in Europe for decades. Acupuncture today is a major form of treatment for nearly one-third of the world's population.

My own experience with acupuncture, including research, teaching and the successful treatment of several thousand patients, has convinced me that it deserves a place in the therapeutic armamentarium of all physicians who treat patients with acute or chronic pain. In my hands, it has been useful with a wide variety of conditions commonly labeled as psychosomatic and has, as well, proved helpful in the management of some psychiatric illnesses. I have, therefore, compiled this text as a means for introducing the subject of modern, physiologic acupuncture in a way that is understandable to graduates of U.S. medical schools. Admittedly, at this time, it is stronger in theory than in fact. Factual matter is not, however, missing and the theories of acupuncture action presented here are well within the realm of acceptable scientific thought.

A few years from now acupuncture will be placed on an even firmer scientific basis. After an existence of several thousand years, it seemed more than timely to present what is now known in such a way that the basic tenets can be incorporated quickly into modern clinical practice.

GEORGE A. ULETT, M.D.

REFERENCES

1. Vieth, I: *The Yellow Emperor's Classic of Internal Medicine.* University of California Press, Berkeley, 1949, p.260.

2. Needham, J., and Lu, Gwei-Pjen: *Celestial Lancets.* Cambridge University Press, Cambridge, 1980, p.427.

CONTENTS

PRINCIPLES AND PRACTICE OF PHYSIOLOGIC ACUPUNCTURE

I

INTRODUCTION

Acupuncture is the most controversial method of non-pharmacological pain control in contemporary medicine. This form of treatment originated in China some 4,000 years ago. It has been of interest in the U.S. for scarcely a decade, although widely used in Europe since early in this century and universally acclaimed for its pain-relieving qualities.

Treatises on traditional acupuncture theory make fascinating reading for one interested in the history of Oriental medicine, but they have little to recommend them to a physician seeking rational direction for assisting his patients in the relief of chronic pain. They fail to explain the possible mechanism of acupuncture treatments in the light of known facts of anatomy and physiology. Yet at this time such alternative, scientific explanations for the action of acupuncture are appearing from many laboratories, including some in Sweden, France, Austria and Canada, as well as in the United States and the People's Republic of China.

The concept of modern medical acupuncture based on experimental and clinical evidence postulates the analgesic effect of acupuncture as essentially the result of sensory interaction in the central nervous system. The pathways for mediation of the pain-inhibiting impulses arising from the point of acupuncture stimulation are believed to be in the extralemniscal system, including the reticular formation, and in the centromedian nucleus of the thalamus. Unit analysis of deep peroneal nerve activity produced by acupuncture of cat anterior tibial muscle demonstrates that such needling activates muscle pressure and stretch receptors, which send afferent volleys over large and medium fibers, (group II and III). The inhibition of pain that occurs has been explained in terms of the "gate theory" of Melzack and Wall. Mounting evidence indicates the importance of the substantia gelatinosa as the area of gate control.

While traditional acupuncturists select from among hundreds of points located on hypothetical meridians, the modern acupuncturist can control pain using only a small number of points. Work from Albert Einstein Medical School in New York has pointed out that some of the most effective acupuncture points coincide with the motor points commonly localized in electromyography. In the treatment of pain, effective points for stimulation may also be selected from within the same dermatome or a neural segment adjacent to the area of pain. Also, electrical stimulation has been found to be more effective than traditional needle twirling, an observation that is substantiated by studies from our own laboratory.

Rapidly gaining scientific support is the hypothesis that, at least in part, acupuncture works through the release of neurotransmitters. Han and collaborators of the Research Group of Acupuncture Anesthesia, Bejing Medical College, have since 1965 steadily accumulated evidence that acetylcholine, serotonin, and endogenous opiate-like substances are all increased through the activation of nerves by means of acupuncture stimulation. These substances, through a facilitating action, increase the acupuncture analgesic effect while their antagonists, including norepinephrine, dopamine, and naloxone, have the opposite effect. Wen and Cheung of Hong Kong reported in 1973 the use of electrically stimulated ear acupuncture for the relief of symptoms of withdrawal from opium addiction. Since then, Wen and collaborators have investigated the effect of electroacupuncture on various biochemical modalities, including B-endorphins, adrenocorticotropic hormone, thyroid-stimulating hormone, and cyclic nucleotides. Researchers at the National Institutes of Health have recently confirmed the release of pain relieving endorphins into the CSF of rats after stimulation of ear acupuncture points.

While a sizeable number of experiments and clinical observations have been reported, much more work is needed to answer the many questions that still exist about acupuncture treatment. There seems little doubt, however, that a more physiologically determined acupuncture-type stimulation can and will play an increasingly important role in the relief of pain.

In this manual we have reviewed evidence in support of a physiological basis for acupuncture. We describe methods for needle application and illustrate examples of motor, trigger point and neurotome area stimulation for the treatment of pain and other conditions. The use of this approach has permitted a rational interpretation of the beneficial results obtained and permitted modification of treatments as necessary on a scientific basis.

Finally in the Appendix we present a brief summary of traditional Chinese acupuncture. This is not essential to our theory but is of historical interest and may be useful to physicians who encounter patients expecting their doctor to be conversant with the terms of classical methodology.

II

PSYCHOLOGICAL VERSUS PHYSIOLOGICAL MECHANISMS—RESEARCH CONSIDERATIONS

Since its introduction into the Western world, there has been much debate as to whether the mechanism of acupuncture is psychological or physiological in nature. Pronouncements were early made by two leading hypnotists: Spiegel (1) and Kroger (2), that acupuncture was a kind of Oriental induction ceremony. This opinion, coming from vast experience with hypnosis had the "halo" effect of strengthening the widespread belief that acupuncture was but a form of hypnosis.

As persons have become more familiar with acupuncture their opinions have changed. Patrick Wall, for example, stated in 1972 (3), "My own belief is that... acupuncture is an effective use of hypnosis." In 1974 (4), after a study tour of China, he retracted that statement. Ronald Katz (5), who reported that a positive response to acupuncture was closely related to a high score on the Hypnosis Induction Profile (HIP), later stated (6), "I have assisted at four operations under acupuncture anesthesia and many more than that under hypnosis. The patients behaved differently. Those under hypnosis are in a tight, self-controlled world, seemingly unaware of what is going on about them. Patients under acupuncture were part of the team, joking, laughing and commenting freely."

My own experience has been similar. Since 1945, I have researched, published, taught and clinically used hypnosis. Until 1970, I knew nothing of acupuncture but when I first became aware of it, I, too, believed it to be a form of hypnosis. My coworkers and I were awarded the first NIH grant to study the relationship between acupuncture and hypnosis. Since then I have studied acupuncture in Japan, China and Europe, have researched, published and taught acupuncture and used it to treat several thousand patients. I am now firmly of the opinion that acupuncture and hypnosis are two different phenomena.

I will not attempt an extensive review of the numerous studies supporting both sides of the question, "Is acupuncture hypnosis?" Reviews by Knox (7) and Lu and Needham (8) cover the subject thoroughly. The latter state that "one cannot deny the importance of a certain measure of suggestion and suggestibility such as is inevitable in all therapies, but that it is a gross misuse of the term 'hypnosis' to cover all aspects of acupuncture treatment." They note that acupuncture has long been an effective part of veterinary medicine in China and that surgery can be accomplished successfully in animals without any question of hypnosis. They conclude that the "vast majority of observers find little in common between acupuncture analgesia and hypnosis." Clinical studies by Moore, *et al.* (9) and Kepes, *et al.* (10) concluded that there was no difference between a classic (real) acupuncture point and a placebo point. However, experimental studies from our laboratory (24) demonstrated differential effects between point and non-point stimulation.

Omura (11), studied 300 patients and included the Spiegel Eyeroll Test. He found those persons with hypnotizability scores above three had a "slightly better" response to acupuncture. Yet more than 50% of people with hypnotizability scores of zero showed beneficial effects of acupuncture. Matsumoto (12), with a similar experience using acupuncture both clinically and experimentally, concludes "...our clinical experiments mitigate against the concept that acupuncture is a form of hyponosis". Others have voiced this same opinion (13,14,15,16). It is recognized that hypnotic induction need not be formal. However, Liao (89) has pointed out that hypnotic induction typically requires prolonged attention of physician to patient whereas with acupuncture this relationship is customarily relatively brief.

As reported in the literature and as discussed later in this book, there are several types of neurophysiologically active acupuncture points including motor points, trigger points and points adjacent to major nerve trunks and nerve plexuses. The use of such different types of point can well be a reason for different experimental results. In some cases the effective points are in close proximity to the site of pain, in other cases quite remote although still in the same neurotome as is the case of LI-4 in the interspace between thumb and first finger, yet useful for dental analgesia. In other cases the point used appears useful for distant effects due to stimulation of a major nerve trunk i.e., the sciatic nerve. This is stimulated by point ST-36 below the knee and has its effect on distant points of the neuraxis presumably through activation of the leg area of the thalamus and in the cortical homunculus. Ear acupuncture (auriculotherapy) has been useful for its stimulation of autonomic fibers with widespread effects on body viscera and hence a usefulness in the treatment of withdrawal symptoms from drug addiction (19).

Some confusion in the literature may also be accounted for by the fact that various authors have used different parameters of acupuncture point stimulation. Thus Andersson (17) has suggested that slow electrostimulation may be specific for acute pain and rapid stimulation for chronic pain. Patterson (20) has suggested that addiction to different drugs may require treatment with different frequencies of electrical ear stimulation. It is our experience that clinical and experimental pain are different phenomena and hence respond differently to acupuncture. Cold pressor pain such as we have utilized in the experimental laboratory, certainly had different characteristics from the chronic pain syndromes that make up the bulk of acupuncture practice. Thus in evaluating different results reported from several experimental laboratories one must consider all of the above possible variables as well as personality, social and environmental differences affecting the populations studied.

In 1975 Goldstein and Hilgard (18), pointed out that while naloxone inhibits the analgesia of morphine and acupuncture, it does not inhibit hypno-analgesia. The endorphin picture as it relates to acupuncture, hypnosis, and pain is far more complex than it originally appeared to be. Yet there is much evidence that polypeptides and other neurotransmitters play important roles here, but differently in those parts of the neuraxis that may relate to acupuncture or hypnosis.

Some have attempted to write off acupuncture as "only" placebo. Certainly placebo plays an important role here as it does in all treatment procedures—perhaps here even stronger than many others due to its special mystique and widespread publicity. Many of the so-called "meridian points" of traditional acupuncture are probably placebo points with mainly historical interest. But as we have demonstrated, even placebo point stimulation can produce some type of physiologic effect. Although initiated by psychological factors, there is now strong evidence (27) that the placebo response utilizes specific neural pathways and thus can serve to augment the physiologic mechanisms of pain modulation by acupuncture.

There have been few studies of the course and nature of the placebo response. We are of the opinion that it accompanies a readiness to respond, based upon strong expectation and hope and that it is seen almost immediately or at least early in the course of treatment. We see such response with some patients receiving acupuncture but these are in the minority. Most of our patients show a gradual improvement developing over a course of treatments and may not show any relief of pain until several treatments have been given. Some of these latter are ones in whom we had anticipated an immediate placebo effect as they came with every expectation of a quick, miracle cure, having read glowing reports in the press and perhaps having seen a television documentary from the People's Republic of China of painless surgery performed under acupuncture analgesia. Despite such strong faith, some such patients have received no benefit from acupuncture or have responded in the more usual manner of gradual relief from pain over a course of eight to twelve treatments.

Delineation of the role of neurophysiology and neurochemistry in producing acupuncture analgesia has been most clearly summarized by Han (21). He showed the similarity of curves of decay from cessation of electrical stimulation which first suggested that some chemical factor was at work. This led to experiments in which cross circulation of both blood and cerebro-spinal-fluid demonstrated that analgesia could be so transferred from one animal to another. Currently this work is directed towards identifying the neurochemicals involved at various brain loci.

Gunn (22), has, in a series of papers, summarized neurophysiological processes whereby spondylosis can produce a vulnerability that may precede painful lesions in almost any neurotome with distant reflections in corresponding myotome, dermatome or sclerotome. He has explained the action of acupuncture utilizing concepts from Cannon's Law of Denervation and the gate theory of Melzack and Wall (23).

Our own work began with a study for locating acupuncture points (24). We found that there were points on the upper extremity, symmetrically located and more or less constant in position from one person to another (Figure 1). These points were a few millimeters in diameter on the skin and differed from the surrounding area by 2-42 millivolts. Since then other investigators have found some such points to be identical with the neurovascular hilus (25).

→

Figure 1. Skin points identified by measurement of resting skin potential. Points are symmetrical on the two extremities and are comparable in location from one person to another and to the acupuncture points shown in the diagram on the right. From Brown, M.L., Ulett, G.A., and Stern, J.A.: Acupuncture loci: Techniques for location. *Amer. J. Chinese Med.*, 1974, 2(1):67-74.

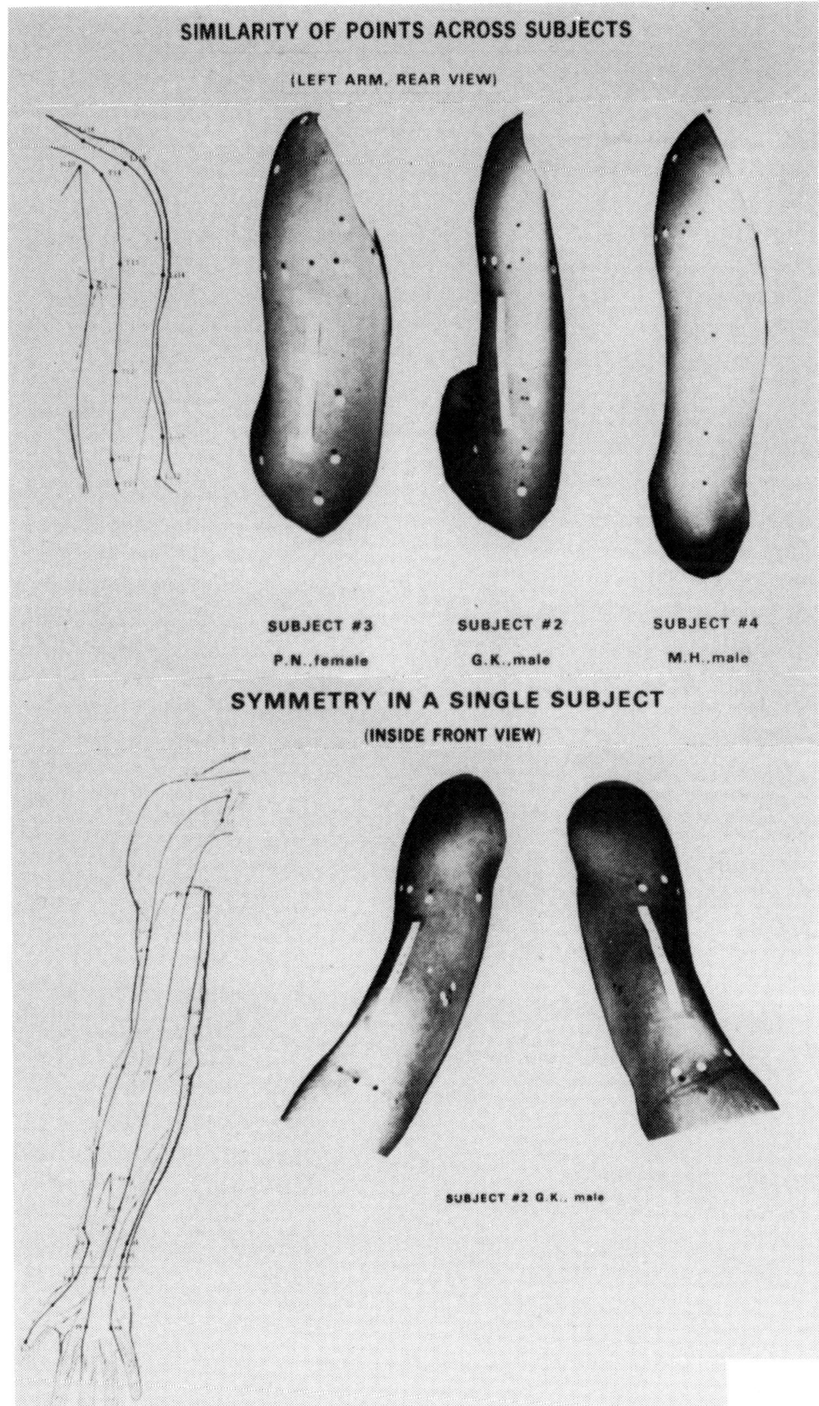
SIMILARITY OF POINTS ACROSS SUBJECTS
(LEFT ARM, REAR VIEW)
SUBJECT #3
P.N., female
SUBJECT #2
G.K., male
SUBJECT #4
M.H., male
SYMMETRY IN A SINGLE SUBJECT
(INSIDE FRONT VIEW)
SUBJECT #2 G.K., male

We also published on the effect of acupuncture on white blood cell counts (26), showing a gradual increase in such response, varying with the degree of stimulation. A slight increase occurred with insertion of the needle alone and the greatest increase with electrical stimulation of the needle. As shown in Figure 2, when the electrical stimulation stopped the white blood cell count fell promptly to the baseline.

Other workers have noted white blood cell changes with acupuncture. Lu and Needham (8), quote the work of Omura and others who relate changes in triglycerides, gamma globulin, ACTH and a host of other blood constituents following acupuncture stimulation. Omura (28) reports changes in the microcirculation as first a constriction followed by dilatation as stimulation continues. We observed changes in skin temperature of the extremities that could result from such effects upon circulation (26).

It is noteworthy that there is a differential of responding with various stimulation intensities. With sufficient intensity of electro-acupuncture, the spread of stimulation through the tissue from a placebo point can activate a nearby neuro-vascular hilus, Golgi organ or nerve plexus. It is also reported that the effect on pain can vary with different parameters of stimulation in terms of wave form or Hertz. Some stimulating equipment available from China allows for changes in wave shape, pulse and train duration, and a frequency selection from 1 to 1,000 Hertz.

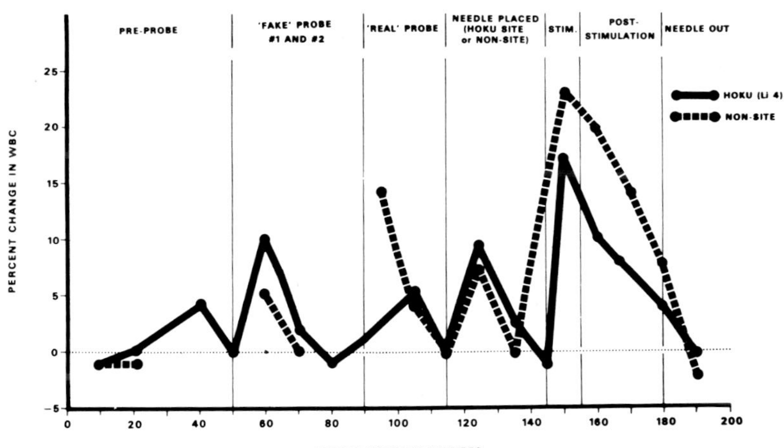

Figure 2. Change in WBC with different intensities of acupuncture stimulation. From Brown, M.L., Ulett, G.A., and Stern, J.A.: The effects of acupuncture on white blood cell counts. *Amer. J. Chinese Med.*, 1974, 2(4):383-398.

The major thrust of our research was to compare the effects of acupuncture and hypnosis on experimental pain (29,30,31,32). We studied 20 healthy male volunteers using cold pressor (water bath) pain, ischemic (tourniquet) pain and the pain of the electrical stimulation used for somato-sensory evoked potentials. We studied the protective effects of 35 minutes of hypnotic suggestion and the insertion of acupuncture needles both at specific and non-specific (placebo) acupuncture loci, both with and without electrical stimulation. These methods were compared to each other, and as well with the administration of morphine sulfate (10 mg.), 5 grains of acetylsalicylic acid (aspirin), 10 mg of diazepam (Valium), 1 and 5 mg of Ketamine/kg and a lactose placebo. Some of the results can be seen in the accompanying figure (Figure 3) showing the effect of different challengers on the intensity of experimental pain.

In summary, our studies found: hypnosis was more effective than electro-acupuncture and morphine sulfate in reducing experimental pain; electrical stimulation of true acupuncture points significantly reduced cold pressor pain while ischemic pain was reduced by both hypnosis and electroacupuncture. We found that the EEG, taken during acupuncture, showed an increase in beta activity while under hypnosis alpha and theta predominated. While our good hypnotic subjects did respond better to both hypnosis and acupuncture, we found that poor hypnotic subjects also responded well to electro-acupuncture.

Electro-acupuncture given at specific acupuncture points was found to be an effective agent for reducing experimental pain. We determined that hypnotic susceptibility does not account for the effectiveness of acupuncture. It was our observation that the analgesic effect of acupuncture was unrelated to anxiety level, subject selection, prior education, suggestion or distraction, such as are generally implicated in pain reduction using methods other than pharmacologic.

In our investigations we also compared the effect of 35 minutes of hypnotic suggestion with 20 minutes of electro-acupuncture stimulation on cold pressor pain in 20 patients who had received clinical acupuncture treatments for relief of chronic low back or knee pain. The patients were divided equally into groups which had experienced good pain relief or a poor result with less than 50% reduction in pain. We found that patients who had done well in treatment i.e., good acupuncture responders, felt less pain with experimental cold pressor stimulation than did those patients who had had a poor clinical result. That is, those who had less clinical pain reduction felt the experimental pain more keenly. In the patients studied, hypnotic susceptibility and response to acupuncture were independent variables. Hypnotic response did not predict acupuncture response.

CHANGES IN SUBJECTIVE EXPERIENCE OF THE SEP STIMULUS INTENSITY ("PAIN")

WITH DIFFERENT PAIN CHALLENGERS

N: 20

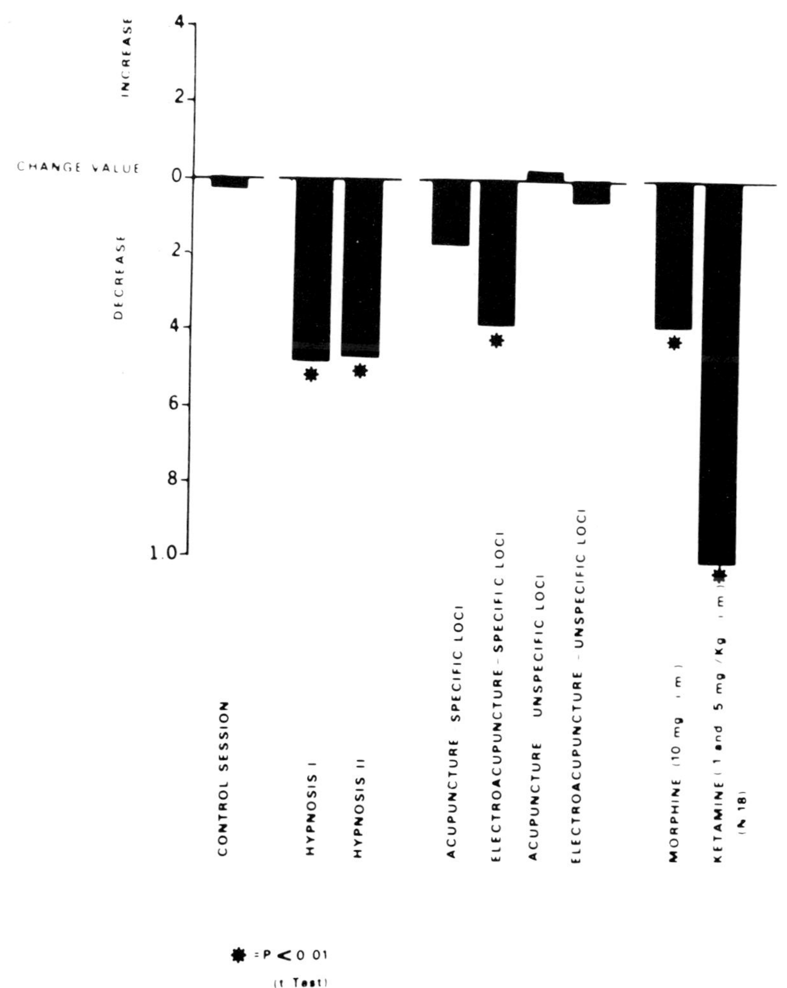

Figure 3. Decrease in pain threshold to experimental pain produced by electrical stimulation of the skin with different pain challengers, including hypnosis and electro-acupuncture. From Saletu, B., Saletu, M., Brown, M.L., Stern, J.A., Sletten, I.W., and Ulett, G.A.: Hypno-analgesia and acupuncture analgesia: A neurophysiologic reality. *Neuropsychobiology*, 1975, 1:218-242.

In clinical practice I have found electro-acupuncture a useful therapeutic tool when employed for the relief of various types of chronic pain (33,39). Almost all of my patients have "worn thin" their placebo response with several other physicians and found even the newest most colorful analgesic capsules to be ineffective for pain relief. Some come in desperation and bear the needles reluctantly. In even this seemingly hopeless group more than 50% obtain some relief from severe disabling pain of long duration.

It has become increasingly clear from the investigations reviewed here that hypnosis and acupuncture act in different ways upon the complex pain mechanisms within the central nervous system. These two methods then are complementary to each other. In some patients where acupuncture has failed hypnosis has proved of some value. In those patients in whom I have recently utilized a combined technique of acupuncture and hypnosis the relief from pain seemed to be exceptionally good.

CONCLUSION

There is sufficient evidence available today to support scientific explanations for the mechanism of the acupuncture effect. It must also be accepted that hypnosis and the placebo response are also effective non-drug means for moderating chronic pain. It is probable that in any given patient with chronic pain all three of these mechanisms may be effective.

III

PAIN MECHANISMS

Acute and chronic pain affect nearly one-half of the population annually. In the U.S. alone the cost is estimated at 85-90 billion dollars a year. Despite the great advances in medical science our efforts to control pain are often ineffectual. For millions of patients chronic pain and suffering continue unabated with severe physical, social and emotional consequences.

Pain is a complex phenomenon involving nociception, pain sensation, suffering and behavioral responses (Figure 5). Pain includes stimulation from the periphery, modulating factors in the substantia gelatinosa of the spinal cord, ascending and descending neural systems, biochemical, physiologic and psychological mechanisms. These are not static, but constantly changing, involving all parts of the nervous system concerned with both sensory and motor systems and, in between, the integrative portion of the central nervous system: subcortical-cortical, paleo-and neocortex, concerned with perceptual, motivational, cognitive, judgemental and affective processes. Kerr has recently summarized the anatomical basis of these pain mechanisms (34).

Anatomically well defined nerves connect all parts of the body, external and internal, with the central nervous system, spinal cord and brain. These peripheral nerves transmit to the central nervous system, for its scrutiny, decision and action, a great variety of impulses. Such impulses travel over fibers of various size. Figure 6 illustrates the makeup of a typical peripheral nerve in terms of representation of fibers of different size. The large myelinated fibers are called A-fibers and are classified according to decreasing size as A-alpha, A-gamma, A-beta and A-delta. B fibers are even smaller in diameter, while C fibers, having no myelin sheath, are the smallest in diameter of all. Large myelinated A-fibers are responsible for efferent, motor impulses from the anterior (ventral) horn cells of the spinal cord to implement the movement of the muscles. Large myelinated A-fibers conduct the proprioceptive impulses that constantly barrage the dorsal horn reporting the movement and position of all body muscles. Large myelinated fibers conduct impulses rapidly, the small myelinated fibers less rapidly, and the smallest unmyelinated C-fibers have the slowest conduction rate of all.

It was early shown by investigators at Washington University in St. Louis (Erlanger, Gasser, Bishop, Heinbecker and O'Leary) that sharp pain was conducted over the finest myelinated (A-delta) fibers while the

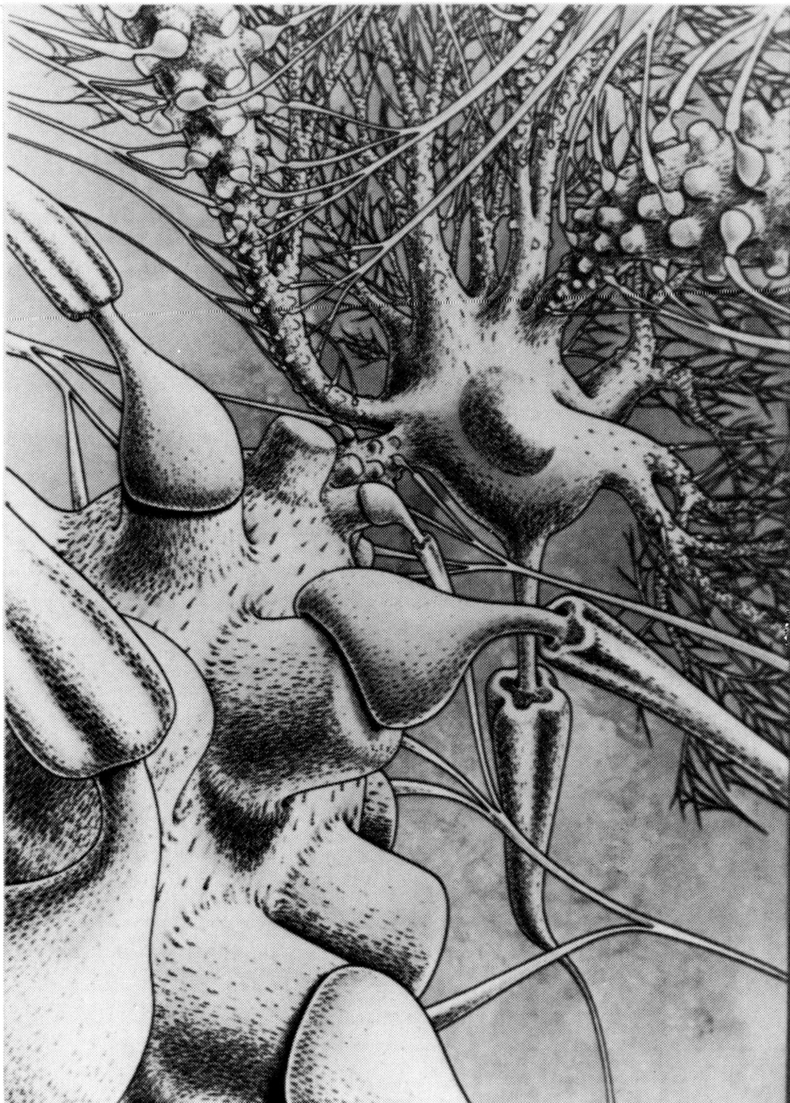

Figure 4. Micro-drawing of typical neuron communication network indicating the complexity of relationships possible in pain perception and pain modulating mechanisms such as acupuncture. (Illustration in brochure from Astra Pharmaceutical Company.)

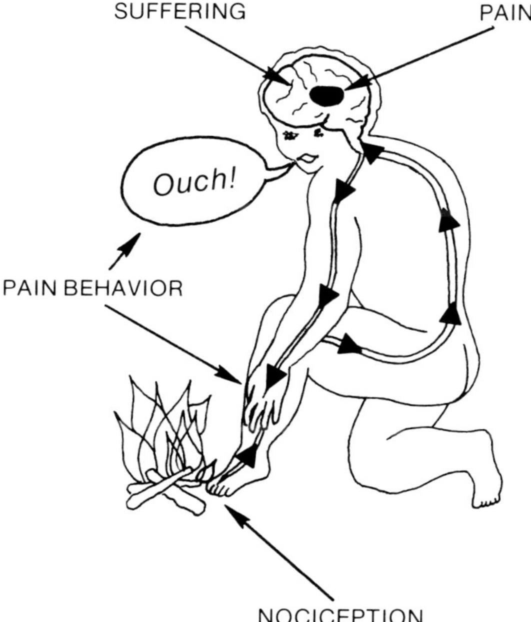

Figure 5. The complexity of the pain phenomenon from the nociceptive stimulus to the behavioral response.

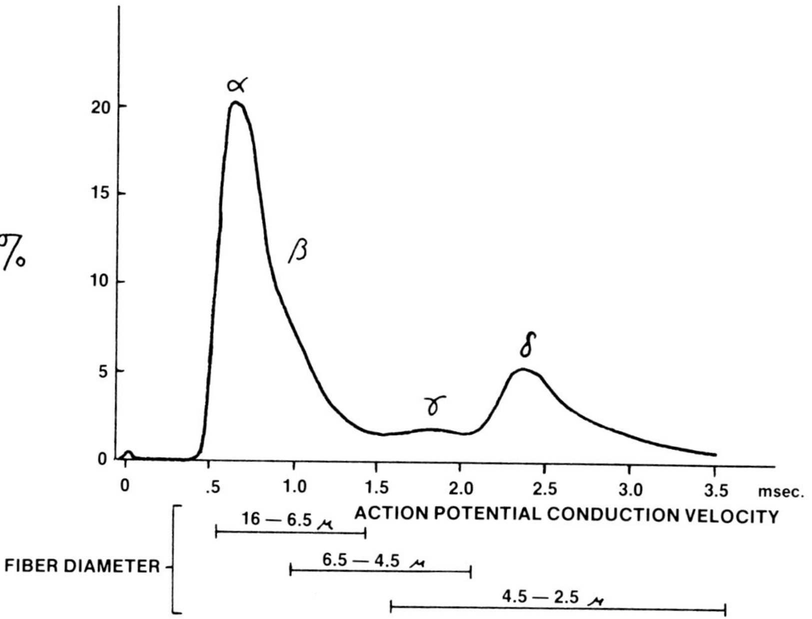

Figure 6. Afferent fiber size representation in typical peripheral nerve.

second pain sensation (dull, aching) was the result of slower conducting, unmyelinated (C) fibers. It was also shown that differentiated receptors were not necessary for the transduction of pain, free nerve endings being sufficient.

These two types of pain have been demonstrated to travel over separate pathways. The sharp first pain travels over the fast conducting oligosynaptic neospinothalamic tract travelling laterally in the spinal cord to reach the thalamus; the other from the anterolateral quadrant of the spinal cord over a polysynaptic paleospinothalamic tract, slow conducting and distributed medially to the reticular core of the brain stem for the second dull, aching pain.

The first type of nociceptor (A-delta) fine medulated fibers are known as high threshold mechanoreceptor afferents which respond only to intensive mechanical stimulation such as when a needle pierces the skin. The second type of nociceptor (C-unmyelinated) nerves are known as polymodal nociceptive and respond to noxious chemicals such as the bradykinens and prostaglandins that are released after tissue injury. Such action of these nerves may account for the long lasting sensation and hyperalgesia following tissue damage.

A. DORSAL HORN PROCESSING

The pain process begins with the all too familiar tissue injury from trauma or disease. This produces stimulation of nociceptive receptors with transmission of the impulses over C-fibers and/or A-delta fibers into the dorsal horn of the spinal cord or its homologue of the trigeminal nerve (Figure 7). These fibers terminate on cells throughout various laminae of the dorsal horn (Figure 8). Cells in Laminae I and V receive the bulk of high threshold input and are involved in pain transmission. It appears that the polymodal nociceptive (pain) fibers and the mechanoreceptive fibers follow quite different courses as they reach the spinal cord. The sorting occurs within 1/2mm of their entrance into the cord substance. Some nociceptive fibers composed of both myelinated and unmyelinated axons distribute in the superficial layers of the dorsal horn (marginal zone Laminae I) and the substantia gelatinosa (Laminae II and III). Unmyelinated fibers are reported as being distributed exclusively in Laminae II. Neurons in the substantia gelatinosa are strategically related to incoming afferents and, as well, to dendrites of deeper Laminae IV and V. Many of the mechanoreceptor fibers (fine medullated), penetrate deeply along the medial aspect of the dorsal horn and then reverse direction to reach the substantia gelatinosa from its ventral surface. In this way synaptic contacts are possible between their afferents and, most, if not all, substantia gelatinosa neurons. These neurons

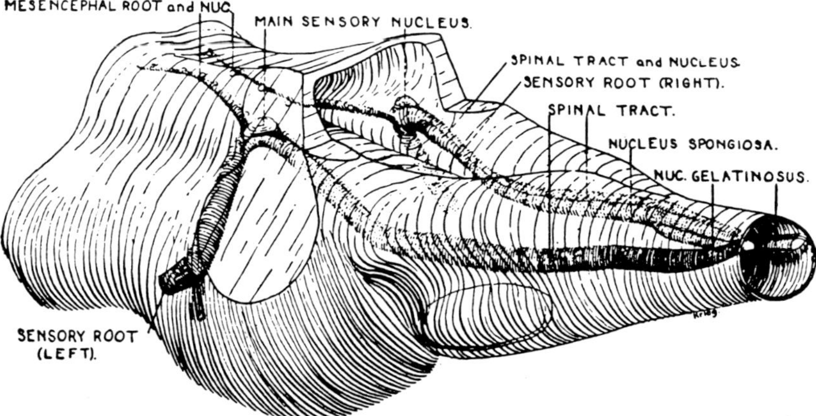

Figure 7. Location of trigeminal, spinal 5th nucelus in brain stem and upper cervical cord. From Krieg, Wendell, J.S.: *Functional Neuroanatomy.* McGraw Hill, New York, Second Edition, 1953.

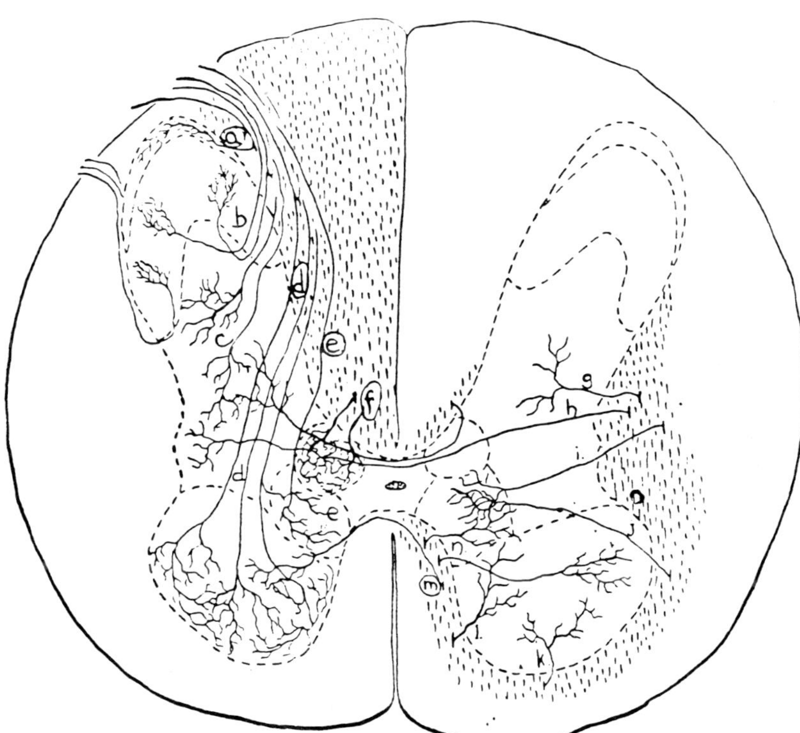

Figure 8. Substantia gelatinosa, (b) site of pain affect input and modulation at spinal cord level. From Krieg, Wendell, J.S.: *Functional Neuroanatomy*. McGraw Hill Book Company, New York, Second Edition, 1953.

then are accessible to activation by both mechanoreceptor and nociceptor afferents. Their axons have been reported to enter the tract of Lissauer and run for distances of up to five segments. This is important for an understanding of how acupuncture needling (mechano-receptor stimulation) can affect pain (nociception), not only within a single segmental level but in adjacent and more widely separated segmental levels as well.

Modulation of pain at the spinal cord level can be explained by a theory of excitatory and inhibitory neurons as follows: a) Marginal neurons receive primary afferent nociceptive input on dendrites in the marginal zone yet also have some deep dendrites which may receive mechanoreceptor input. b) Presumed inhibitory input from gelatinosa neuron ends on their soma. c) Descending systems from the brain stem terminate fairly equally on both soma and proximal dendrites. An inhibitory feedback circuit is provided which is activated by stimulation of mechanoreceptive afferents (as by needleprick stimulation, skin rubbing, etc.). These afferents activate enormous numbers of gelatinosa neurons whose terminals provide post-synaptic inhibition of marginal neurons.

The role of various neurotransmitters in this area has yet to be fully elucidated. It seems clear, however, that a main transmitter of pain impulses is substance P. This is present in the neurons of the substantia gelatinosa and is blocked by enkephalin release. Such enkephalin release may well be accomplished by modulation pathways from supra-segmental structures activated by ascending nociceptive impulses.

B. ASCENDING PATHWAYS

The nociceptive input undergoes integrative processing in the spinal cord dorsal horn or the trigeminal spinal nucleus. The modified message is then relayed on both crossed and ipsilateral axons of the marginal neurons of Laminae V and VI. These spinal afferent tracts ascend in the anterior lateral quadrant of the spinal cord and terminate at various levels of the neuraxis. One of these tracts is the spinothalamic which projects to the ventrobasal thalamus, intralaminar thalamic nuclei and posterior thalamus.

Another tract in the anterior lateral quadrant is the spinoreticular pathway. A majority of its fibers terminate in the ventromedial part of the bulbar reticular formation, nucelus gigantocellularis. Some of the cells here, in turn, project to the mesencephalic reticular formation and the intralaminar thalamic nuclei. Other spino-reticular afferent tracts project directly to the mesencephalic reticular formation and the periaqueductal gray substance in the area of the mesencephalic-diencephalic junction. This area lies medial to the medial geniculate body. It is concerned with nociceptive input while a third of the magnocellular subnucelus of the medial geniculate nucleus appears more concerned with mechanoreceptor and auditory input. An area lateral and ventrolateral to the peri-aquiductal gray, named the nucleus cuneoformis has been shown to contain neurons which respond selectively to nociceptive stimuli.

At the thalamic level the neospinothalamic system terminates throughout the ventro-postero-lateral nucleus, overlapping with the termination of the medial lemniscus. Another portion of the neospinothalamic system distributes to the para-fascicular, intralaminar and paralaminar nuclei. Chang (42) found that electrical stimulation of some acupuncture points would inhibit the pain response in neurons at the nucelus para-fasciularis and nucleus centralis lateralis of the thalamus. It is important to note that a major part of the paleospinothalamic system converges again with the neospinothalamic input at the intralaminar nuclei projecting as it does from periaqueductal gray and nucleus cuneiformis.

It has been shown that in addition to the well known termination of nonnociceptive modulators in the ventro-postero-lateral nucleus, approximately one-third of the neurons of this nucleus can be activated by noxious stimuli. Thus, in the thalamus, as well as in the dorsal horn of the spinal cord, both noxious and non-noxious modalities are present in a variable admixture permitting the ready inter-communication of impulses, so important in explaining the modulation of pain by non-pain stimuli. Melzack and Melinkoff (43) raised the pain threshold by stimulation of the cat's midbrain reticular formation. The time course paralleled that seen with acupuncture analgesia in humans. From this they postulated activation of discrete reticular sites which in turn exerted an inhibitory effect on somatic transmission from selective body regions. They felt that such a mechanism could account for the production of analgesia in areas distant from the point of acupuncture stimulation.

While this widespread distribution of nociception renders surgical control of pain difficult and uncertain it offers an explanation of how peripheral stimulation, as by acupuncture can by reaching distant areas of the neuraxis, modulate pain at several levels and in multiple areas of the brain. Superficial skin stimulation and needle-prick can, thus, modulate noxious stimuli through a blocking influence of faster acting A-delta (mechanoreceptor) fibers on cells activated by nociceptive afferents at both segmental and suprasegmental levels. It seems likely, moreover, particularly at the thalamic level, that noxious impulses could come under the influence of afferent stimuli generated by electro-acupuncture of the major muscle afferent tracts activated by needle placement in the neuro-vascular hilae. It has been postulated by Gunn (22), that needling may also be effective with placement near flower spray endings and near Golgi organs at tendon junctions (Figure 9).

Andersson and co-workers (44), point out that there is no reason to believe that acupuncture activates other than known physiological mechanisms. The sensation of "teh chi" (swelling, drawing, soreness and numbness) is said to be essential for obtaining the therapeutic effectiveness of acupuncture. This sensation arises from stimulation of A-delta fibers and is, thus, mainly obtained from muscle nerves. It was concluded by Andersson (45), that stimulation of muscle afferents at intensities activating high threshold nerves is important in producing acupuncture effects. The afferents are also activated during strong muscular activity and the above workers have studied the effect on pain threshold of free running activity in wheels by hamsters and rats. Such activity produced a long lasting, nalaxone-reversible increase in pain threshold that correlated with the amount of running. The authors suggest that stimulation of such muscle afferent activity during exercise, such as jogging, could produce a similar change in the central nervous system of humans.

Although there is not yet evidence to support it, we have pondered the role of the proprioceptive afferents which are also ubiquitous and stimulated strongly by the muscle contractions produced by such needle placement at motor points. Although there are alternative explanations for the "high" that occurs with jogging (46), it may well be that these play companion or augmenting roles in finally effecting neurotransmitter mechanisms. Jogging and physical exercise have been proposed as a means for the treatment of mild depression. Acupuncture has been similarly used. In both instances, muscle afferents are involved. Thus, as we shall later elaborate, effective acupunture points are those among the traditional meridian locations that coincide in location with or are situated near motor points (neuro-vascular hilae).

Such considerations lead logically to a concept of pain that is far broader than that of simply signaling only tissue injury. Psychiatrists have long considered deep depression to be one of the most "painful" of illnesses. Such patients are engulfed in a suffering that often includes an awareness of dysfunction in body organ systems. In patients with chronic pain one often finds severe dysphoria (anxiety and depression).

Acupuncture may, thus, have a wider usefulness than modulating the noxious impulses that arise from injury to peripheral tissue. With access of the acupuncture stimulus to both cortical and subortical structures it can well affect cranial nerve nuclei including the vagus, and also have an

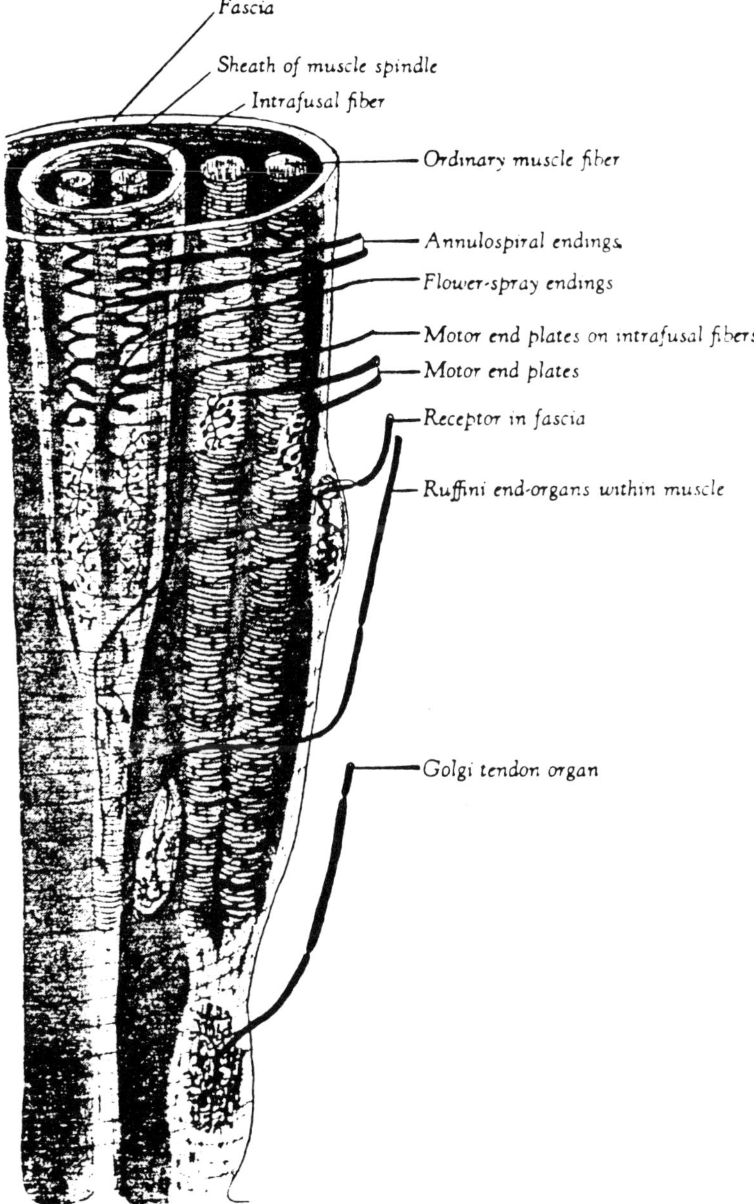

Figure 9. Diagram of flower spray and Golgi endings at tendon junctions. From Krieg, Wendell J.S.: *Functional Neuroanatomy*. McGraw Hill Book Company, New York, Second Edition, 1953.

influence upon the hypothalamus with its control of hormonal and vegetative functions. Pomeranz (47), found in hypophysectomized mice that acupuncture did not produce analgesia in the absence of the pituitary, again indicating the interdependence of neural and hormonal mechanisms.

C. CORTICAL LEVEL

Noxious stimuli act not only at spinal cord and subcortical levels but as well gain ready access to consciousness. The extent of their recognition as unpleasant and the quality and intensity of their emotional consequence, depends upon previous pain experiences, the cultural background, age, sex and the significance of the present situation to the individual. The threshold of pain apparently varies from day-to-day and even hour-to-hour. It is influenced by many environmental factors and, as well, by the circadian tide of hormones which alters the level of various neurotransmitter substances. These influences play upon both cortical and subcortical structures which in turn modulate ascending somato-sensory information through descending pathways terminating on the dorsal horn neurons. Corticofugal pathways from somato sensory cortex can inhibit dorsal horn cells that are activated by low threshold stimulation (tactile), but not noxious stimuli. Pathways descending from the raphe magnus, periaqueductal gray and surrounding tegmentum can inhibit dorsal horn cells that are activated specifically by noxious input.

A major contribution to an understanding of the role of cortex in pain mechanisms comes from the laboratory of Sven Andersson in Gőteborg, Sweden (48,49,50,51). He and his associates working with tooth pulp stimulation in the cat ascertained that information interpreted as pain reaches the cortex via multiple paths with at least two major components. One, a noxious stimulus activates cells diffusely with bilateral thalamic and cortical distribution. These impulses travel in thalamocortical pathways with fibers terminating predominantly in superficial lamina and give long lasting excitatory potentials. The other part of the response has properties similar to that evoked by stimulation of contralateral cutaneous afferents and is mediated via thalamo-cortical fibers arising in the specific thalamic nuclei and terminating in lamina IV of the sensory cortex in a topographical fashion permitting localization of the stimuli in the sensory homunculus of the cortex (Figure 10). A similar projection of fibers has been demonstrated by Chatrian (53). Work has been reported from China (52) where stimulation of the cervical cutaneous nerve and dental pulp in animals was shown to evoke potentials in the sensory cortex. Such potentials could be suppressed by stimulation of

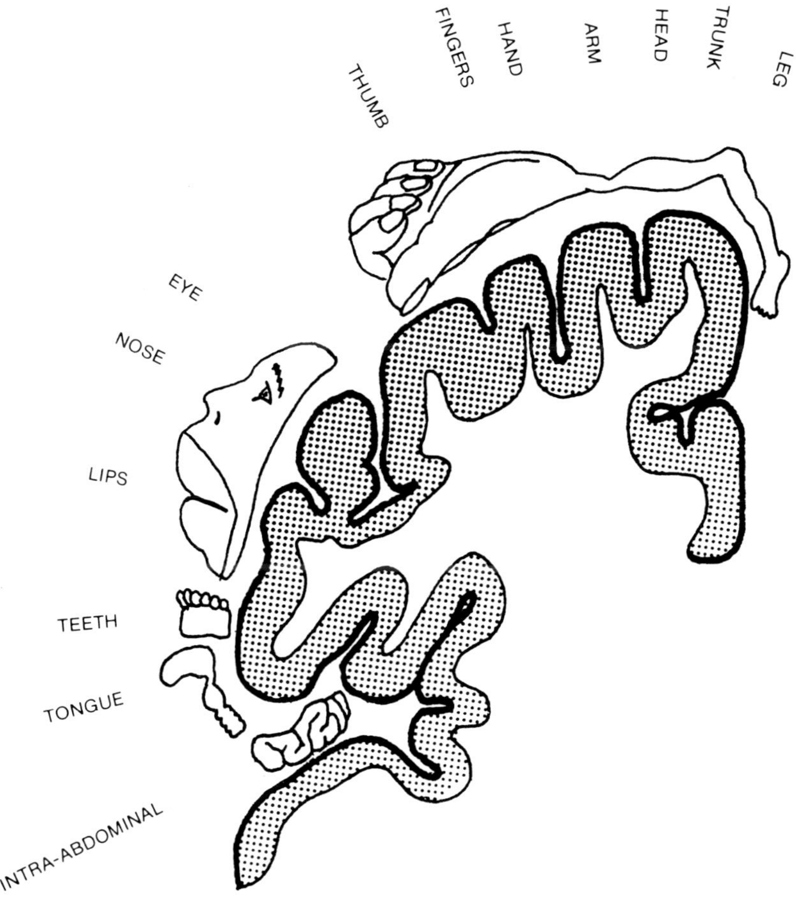

Figure 10. Sensory homunculus of the cerebral cortex.

the acupuncture point LI-4. The widespread nature of the pain response has also been confirmed by an increased cerebral blood flow over large regions of the cortex after a noxious stimulus (54).

It is hypothesized that these two components may underlay respectively the localization and aversive pathways that signal pain and are subjected to inhibitory control at different levels. Such control systems both prevent the sensation of pain, modulate the nervous activity evoked by noxious stimuli (acute pain) and, as well, effect a diminution of chronic pain.

Segmental inhibition can be produced by peripheral stimulation as described under the concept of a dorsal horn gating mechanism. Supraspinal control of the gate mechanism is produced by descending mechanisms from the midbrain and cortex. At least one of these systems seems to have endorphin as a transmitter. This is apparently the system activated by acupuncture since pain relief and increased pain threshold, such as produced by low frequency electrical stimulation or manipulation of needles, can be reversed by naloxone (55).

D. NEUROPHARMACOLOGICAL FACTORS

Basic to any understanding of behavioral neurochemistry is the assumption that certain substances, neuro-regulators, play a key role in the communication among nerve cells. These are divided into two types: those that convey information between adjacent nerve cells (neurotransmitters), and those that amplify or dampen neuronal activity (neuromodulators). Table I lists some of the compounds which have been so classed.

The idea of chemicals being involved in neuronal communication goes back to 1904 and a succession of discoveries since that time pointing first to acetylcholine (ACh), and later to epinephrine, norepinephrine, dopamine, GABA, serotonin and others. Important for the study of neuroregulation in pain was independent demonstration by several groups (56,57,58) in 1973 of opioid receptors in the central nervous system. These receptors are binding sites on neuronal membranes through which all opiate agonists exert their pharmacological action. Opiate antagonists (like naloxone), on the other hand, are able to reverse and block the pharmacological effects of opiate agonists by competitive inhibition at the receptor.

In 1975, Hughes (59), isolated two opiate peptides, methionine-enkephalin and leucine-enkephalin. Subsequently, it was found that the methionine-enkephalin in amino acid sequence also appeared in B-lipotropin and its COOH-terminal 31 amino acid now called B-endorphin.

TABLE I

SOME POSSIBLE CNS REGULATORS

Dopamine
Epinephrine
Norepinephrine
Tyramine
Phenylethylamine
Dimethoxyphenylethylamine (DMPEA)
Serotonin (5-hydroxytryptamine)
Tryptamine
Dimethyltryptamine (DMT)
5-Hydroxydimethyltryptamine (bufotenin)
Acetylcholine
Histamine
Gamma-Aminobutyric acid (GABA)
Glycine
Taurine
Purine
Aspartate
Glutamate
Prostaglandins
Corticosteroids
Estrogens
Testosterone
Thyroid hormone
Enkephalins
B-Endorphin
Substance P
Somatostatin
Angiotensin
Luteinizing hormone releasing hormone (LHRH)
Vasoactive intestinal polypeptide (VIP)
Adrenocorticotropic hormone (ACTH)
Thyroid releasing hormone (TRH)
Sleep factor delta

Both the enkephalins and B-endorphin were found to produce analgesia in man following intracerebral injections.

These compounds called opiate peptides, as well as the opiates are felt to induce analgesia in three possible ways: 1) by inhibiting afferents in the dorsal horn, 2) by inhibiting somato-sensory pathways at supraspinal levels and 3) by activating descending inhibitory pathways.

The peri-aqueductal gray substance is high in opiate binding sites. This includes the medial brain stem structures extending from the rostral portions of the fourth ventricle along the cerebral aqueduct and into regions surrounding the caudal portions of the third ventricle and also a more caudally located region of the nucleus reticularis gigantocellularis.

On stimulation this area is consistently effective in producing analgesia. The mechanism may either be direct neuronal excitation or the inhibition of a tonic inhibitory process.

Mayer (55), showed that narcotic microinjection into the peri-aqueductal grey substance inhibits response of spinal cord "wide dynamic range" neurons to nociceptor stimuli. Those dorsal horn cells that are not responsive to noxious stimuli are unaffected by such narcotic injection. This control through stimulation of nerves by the opiate-like substance descends by way of the dorsal funiculus of the spinal cord (Figure 11).

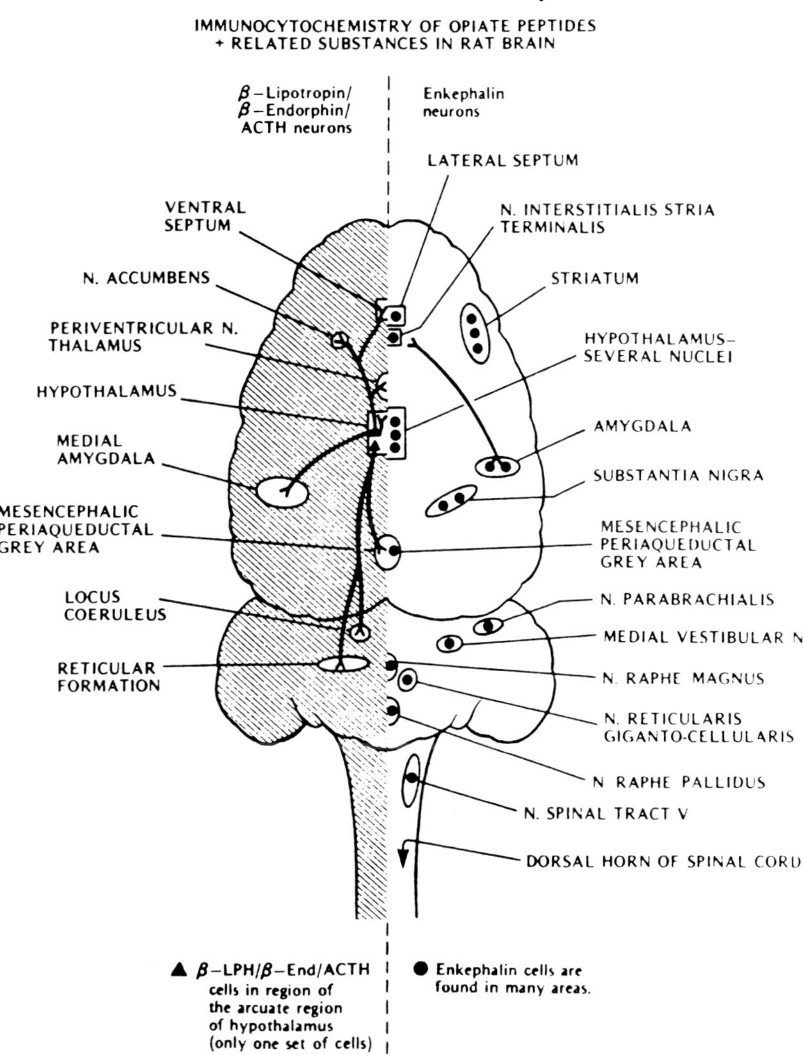

Figure 11. Endogenous, opiate localization in rat brain. From Barchas, J.D., Akil, H., Elliott, G.R., Holman, R.B., and Watson, S.J.: Behavioral neurochemistry: Neuroregulators and behavioral states. *Science*, 1978, 200:964-973. Copyright 1978, by the American Association for the Advancement of Science.

Serotonin is also involved in narcotic analgesia via the midbrain ascending serotonin systems (Figure 12), or the descending medullary system. Increasing serotonin levels directly by intraventricular injection or by systemically administered 5-HTP (5-hydroxytryptamine) will potentiate morphine analgesia. A similar effect occurs with low level stimulation of the dorsal raphe nucleus.

Yao, Andersson and Thorel (44), reported evidence that the central serotonin system and endorphin system, as well, are both involved in depressor response effective for slowing the pulse, decreasing the blood pressure, and inhibiting splanchnic activation after acupuncture-like stimulation of the sciatic nerve. It is of interest that the effect was more pronounced in hypertensive than in normo-tensive rats with the amount of decrease proportional to the initial hypertensive level. This is in keeping with the widespread belief that acupuncture produces a return to homeostatic levels when the physiology is disordered and has a lesser effect when applied to normals. This is one of the mechanisms serving as a basis for the use of acupuncture in the treatment of conditions other than pain.

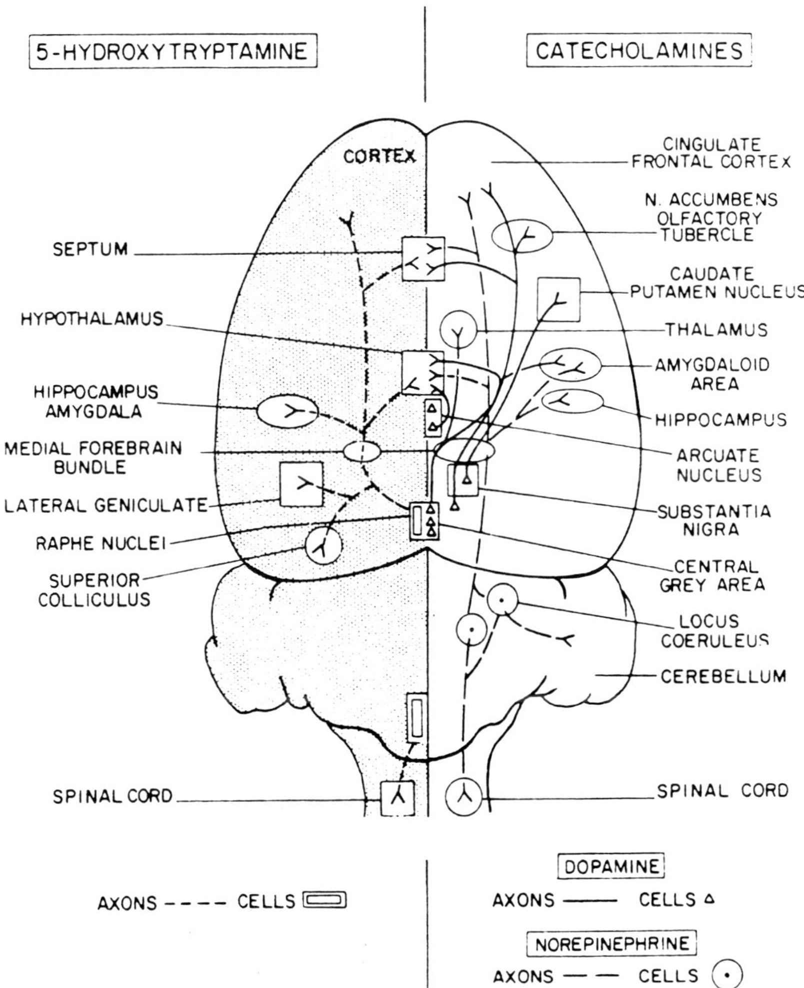

Figure 12. Dopaminergic, noradrenergic and serotinergic pathways in rat brain. From Barchas, J.D., Akil, H., Elliott, G.R., Holman, R.B., and Watson, S.J.: Behavioral neurochemistry: Neuroregulators and Behavioral stress. *Science*, 200:964-973, 1978. Copyright 1978, by the American Association for the Advancement of Science.

Evidence also exists in support of the belief that catecholamines play a role in narcotic analgesia. Thus, 5-HT depletion has been shown to reduce narcotic analgesia while norepinephrine depletion or receptor blockade potentiate it. Norephinephrine, given intravenously, blocks morphine action, while 5-HT, given in the same manner, potentiates it (Figure 13).

Supporting evidence for the release in the brain of an endogenous substance with opiate-like activity as a function of acupuncture, is the demonstration that acupuncture analgesia in humans is reversible by naloxone (60). In similar tests of hypnotically induced analgesia, naloxone had no such antagonistic effects (61,62). Because segmental withdrawal reflexes were suppressed however it appeared that hypnosis did modulate a descending antinociceptive pathway. This pathway however appeared to be one in which opiate-like substance seemed not to be involved.

It is also of interest that analgesia can result from painful and stressful manipulations. This includes such stress as foot shock, cold water swim, injection of hypertonic saline and exposure to a hot plate. This clearly indicates that the phenomenon of pain can be modulated by techniques that involve different pathways using different chemical transmitters thus suggesting the possible augmentation of pain control by the simultaneous use of several different techniques. It is felt that such analgesia comes about by descending influences on both opiate and non-opiate analgesia systems.

Mayer (55) postulates that certain stressors produce analgesia by activating the "opiate analgesia system." He feels that the common factor is a relatively extended exposure to strong somato-sensory stimuli such as that produced by acupuncture electro-stimulation.

SUMMARY

In summary there are, then, alternative central mechanisms for producing analgesia. They result in a selective suppression of nociception and do not produce generalized somato-sensory deficits. Stimulation of non-opiate related systems could partly explain why stimulus produced analgesia is only partially reversed by naloxone and in some animals naloxone has no analgesic effect. Thus, any pathway activated by stimulation must ultimately be classified as narcotic or non-narcotic. Stimulation, as by acupuncture, may involve activation of more than one such system.

With stimulus produced analgesia, the analgesic effect persists well beyond the actual period of stimulation. However, research is necessary

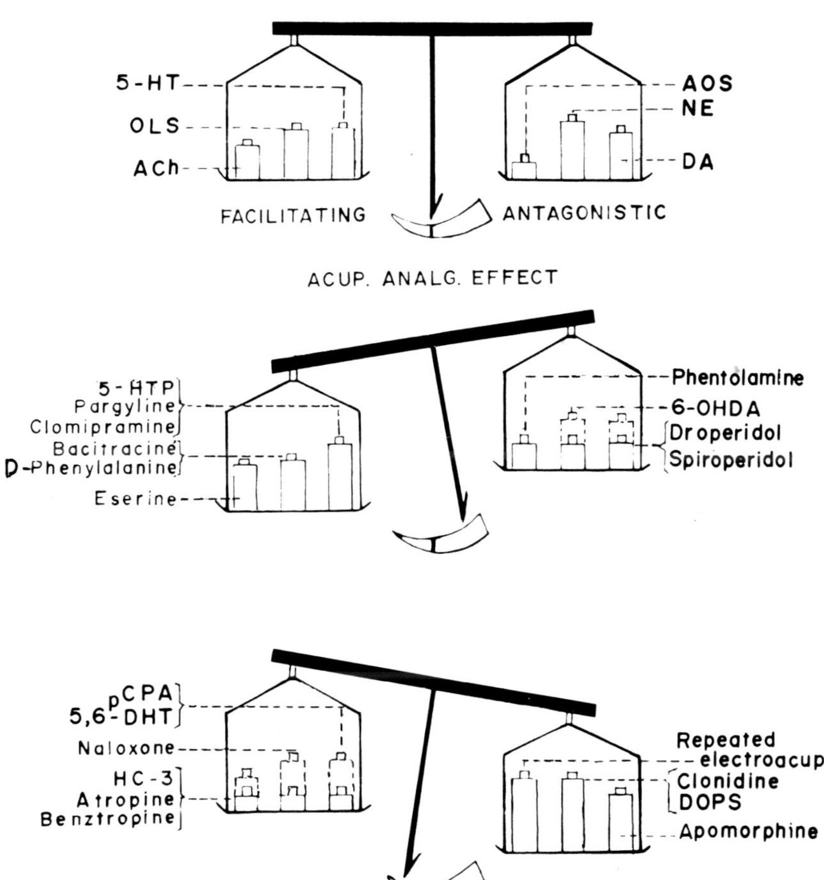

Figure 13. Illustrating increases and decreases in the acupuncture analgesic effect with alterations in the functional activity of central neurotransmitters. From Han, C.S., Tang, J., Jen, M.F., Zhou, A.F., Fan, S.G., and Qio, X.C.: The role of central neurotransmitters in acupuncture analgesia. Private Publication. *Research Group of Acupuncture Anesthesia.* Peking, People's Republic of China.

to establish the most effective parameters of stimulation and to test for a cummulative build-up of analgesia as, for example, with successive acupuncture treatments.

It is known that there are individual differences in pain threshold. This threshold also varies with the time of day, being highest in the morning when the level of endogenous opiates is still high from the circadian rhythm of hormonal secretions. Pain threshold is also modified by many external influences. All of these factors must be taken into consideration as one assesses the results of any method of pain modulation, including acupuncture stimulation.

This chapter has outlined the anatomical and biochemical basis for the production of analgesia. Thus it is shown that there is adequate rationale and scientific basis for mechanisms of acupuncture produced analgesia. As we shall see more clearly in the next section, acupuncture probably works not by one such mechanism alone but by several modes of action.

IV

ACUPUNCTURE AND PAIN

Today there is little doubt that the acupuncture effect is a neurophysiologic phenomenon. Only those with a strong personal commitment to traditional Chinese medicine and a strong belief in occult phenomena (63) hold otherwise. Contemporary Chinese physiologists (64) have demonstrated a neuronally mediated rise in pain threshold from stimulation of the peripheral acupuncture points. This phenomenon was not abolished by vascular occlusion of the limb, however, the analgesic effect was abolished when the nerve was anesthetized by procaine. Work from Sweden (17), our own laboratory (30) and from Canada (65), has indicated that acupuncture needling can raise the pain threshold and that this procedure is more effective when electrical stimulation is added.

The fact that some acupuncture (meridian) points were more effective than others and that "placebo" (non-meridian) points had any effect upon pain threshold seemed puzzling at first. Several explanations, however, are now forthcoming. In the first place not all of the historically designated acupuncture points lie in or near motor points or neural structures. Also, in some instances, the "placebo" needle may turn out to be inadvertently placed in or near a motor point, close to a nerve trunk or tendon end organ. If electrical stimulation is used, proximity is all that is necessary for electrical stimulation spreads through the tissue to produce more remote effects. And, finally, as Stewart, et al have shown (66), as long as the placebo point is located within the same dermatome some increase in pain threshold may be achieved. In all such cases, the needle "pique" through the skin can effectively stimulate A-delta fibers whose impulses can thus block the more slowly conducted nociceptive messages of the C-fibers.

In support of the above and in keeping with the anatomy and neurochemistry previously discussed is the "gate theory" of Melzack and Wall (23). Noordenbos (67) had earlier studied cases with post-herpetic neuralgia in which nerve biopsy specimens showed a preferential loss of large myelinated fibers. Thus it was generalized that pain results from a consequential loss of inhibition that is normally provided by these large fibers. It is now known however that large fiber loss is not necessarily followed by pain. Alteration in sensory input dependent upon nerve fiber size is not sufficient alone to explain the production of pain. However, the theory still holds that the transmission of information about the injury from the periphery to the central nervous system is under the control of or influenced by peripheral afferents. Descending impulses play a role as well. Thus the "gate control theory" (Figure 14), as postulated by Melzack and Wall (23) and later reformulated by Wall (68) states: 1) Information about the presence of injury is transmitted to the central nervous system by the peripheral nerves. Small diameter A-delta and C-fibers respond only to injury while others with lower thresholds increase their discharge frequency if the stimulus reaches noxious levels. 2) Cells in the spinal cord or fifth nerve nucleus that are excited by their injury signals are also facilitated or inhibited by other peripheral nerve fibers that carry information about innocuous events. 3) Descending control systems originating in the brain modulate the excitability of the cells that transmit information about injury. 4) Thus the brain receives messages about injury by way of a gate controlled system that is influenced by (a) injury signals and (b) other types of afferent impulses by both ascending and descending control.

The importance of such a gating mechanism located in the substantia gelatinosa of the spinal cord as initially proposed has gained much support with recommended modifications as research upon the anatomy and neurochemistry of this region continues. Of equal or perhaps even greater importance, however, are similar gating mechanisms at higher brain stem levels (Figure 15). The important work of Chang (69) has

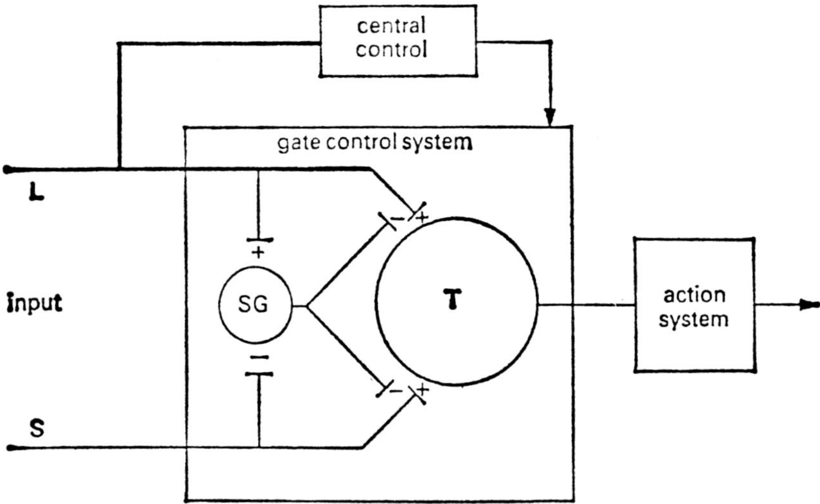

Figure 14. Schematic diagram of the gate-control theory of pain mechanisms. From Melzack, R., and Wall, P.: Pain mechanisms: A new theory. *Science*, 150:971-73, 1965. Copyright 1965, by the American Association for the Advancement of Science.

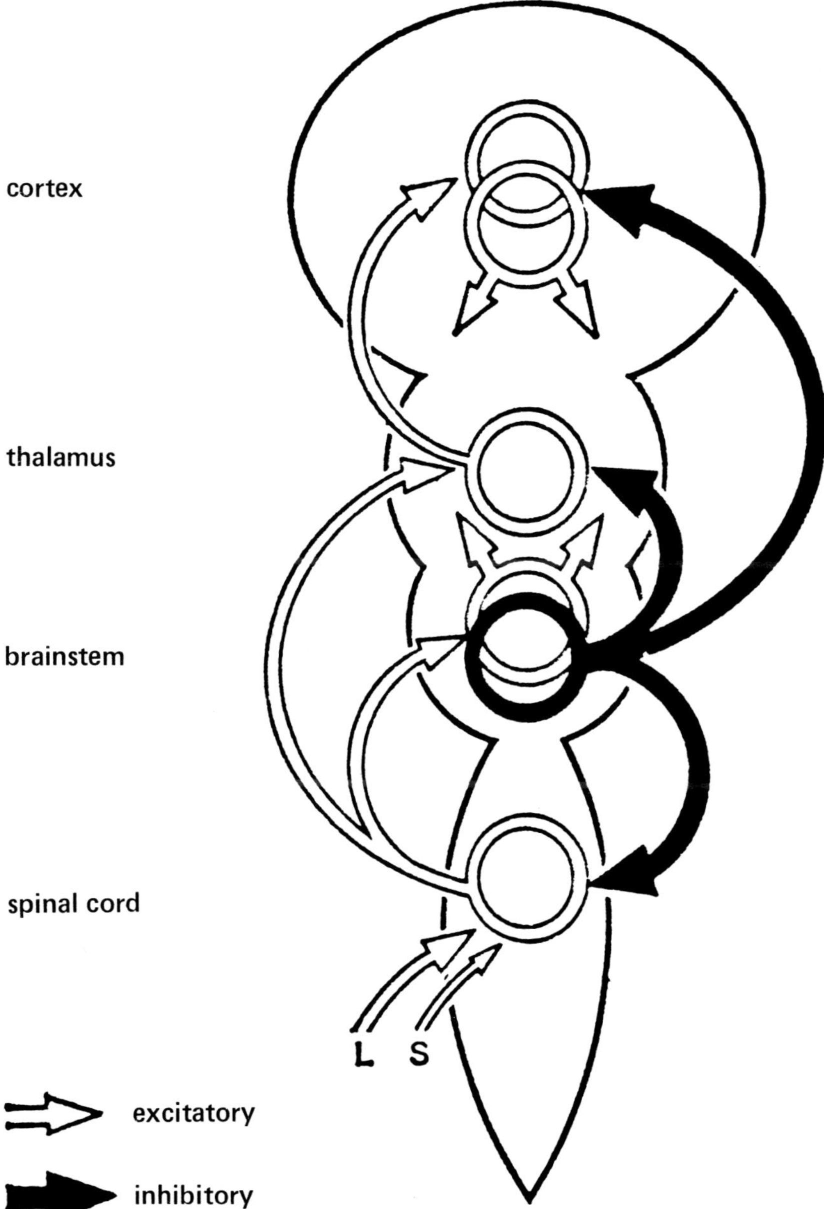

Figure 15. Schematic diagram of central biasing mechanisms "higher level gate." From Melzack, R.: Phantom limb pain. *Anesthesiology*, 35(4):407, 1971.

emphasized thalamic gating mechanisms located particularly in the nucleus parafasciculus and nucleus centralis lateralis. He believes that (under ordinary conditions) these thalamic pain centers are under continuous inhibitory control by incoming sensory impulses. This has been likened to a kind of "normal beneficial jamming of received messages." While under barrage from some noxious stimulation, disinhibition occurs and hyperalgesia ensues. This is one mechanism of intractible central pain. Cells in these nuclei may be made to fire rhythmically in response to noxious stimuli. Such pain response is abolished by the administration of morphine, by electro-acupuncture and by pinching acupuncture points at the Achilles' tendon in animal models.

Another important area in the pain pathway is the raphe magna-cellularis of the medulla. This area could well be important in the production of analgesia in viscero-somatic reflex activities such as the induction of pain by traction upon the mesenteric attachment of abdominal viscera. The proximity of this brain stem area to the nucleus of the vagus nerve suggests a possible mechanism for the alleviation of visceral pain by electro-acupuncture stimulation with needles placed in the concha of the ear, an area innervated by the vagus nerve.

The effectiveness of acupuncture points distant from the site of pain has long seemed a mysterious part of acupuncture manipulation. It has now however been demonstrated that the firing of pain sensitive neurons in the spinal trigeminal nucleus of the medulla produced by electrical stimulation of the alveolar nerve of the dental pulp in cats has been completely suppressed by electro-acupuncture not only at acupuncture points ST-3 on the cheek, but also by LI-4 on the paw. This phenomenon is explained by the fact that modifying impulses from the paw travel via the brachial plexus to segments of the spinal cord in the cervical region. As we have seen these can course upward for several segments for an easy overlap with fibers that similarly descend from the spinal trigeminal nucleus. Experiments such as this give support to our belief that it is important, for pain suppression by acupuncture, to use the principle of placing the modulating stimulus either within the same neurotome from which the focus of pain is arising, and/or, in addition, in areas whose neurotomes lie adjacent to the one involved. Such a segmental approach is basic to successful treatment by acupuncture. Figure 16 shows neurotome distribution of the human body.

That a similar suppression of trigeminal spinal tract neurons has been described from stimulation of ST-36 in the tibial area of the cat's hind limb illustrates that ascending spinal impulses can also influence supraspinal gate mechanisms. On theoretical grounds one would infer that

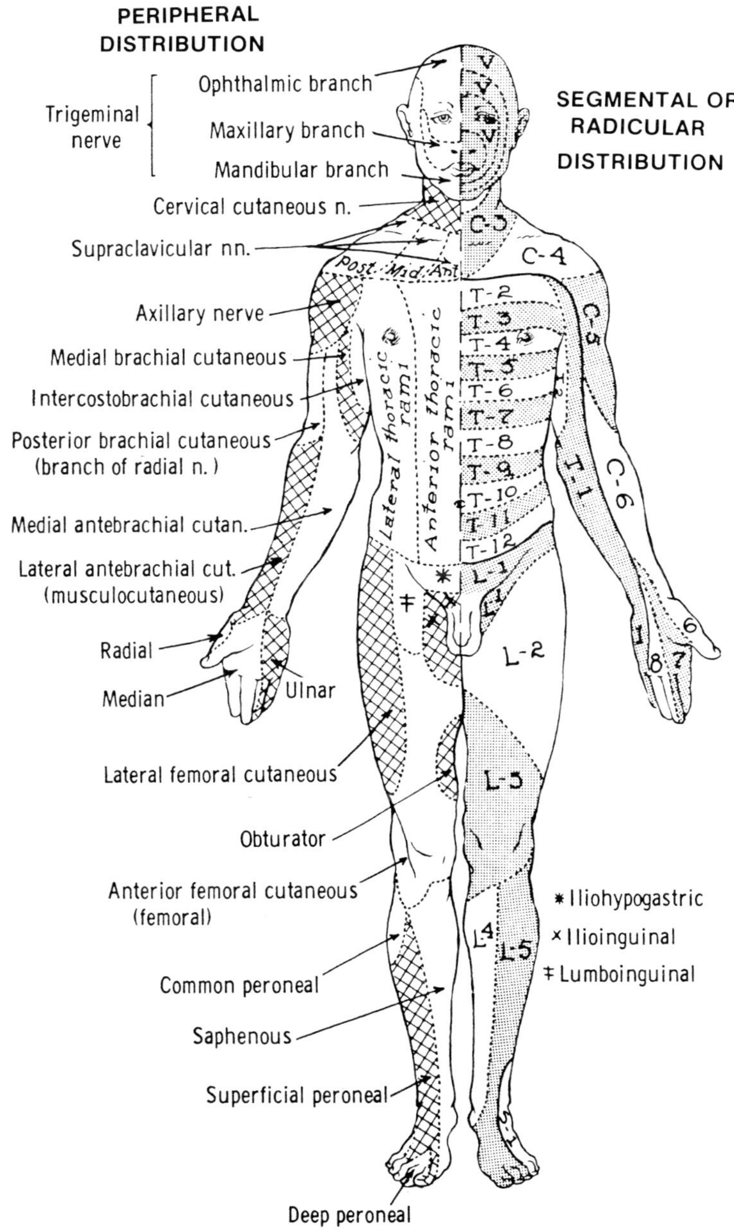

Figure 16. Neurotome distribution on the human body. From McDonald, J.J., Green, J.R., and Lange, J.: *Correlative Neuroanatomy.* Third Edition, 1938. University Medical Publishers, Palo Alto, Ca.

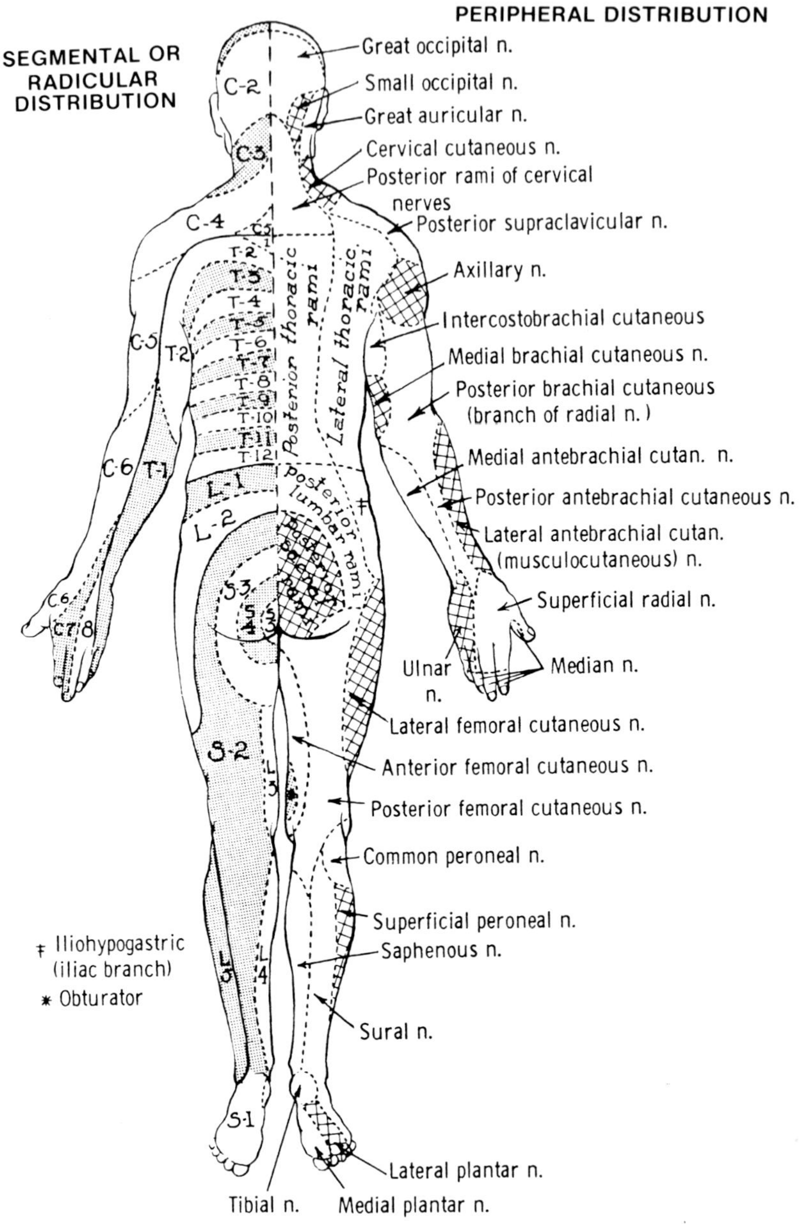
PERIPHERAL DISTRIBUTION
SEGMENTAL OR RADICULAR DISTRIBUTION
Great occipital n.
Small occipital n.
Great auricular n.
Cervical cutaneous n.
Posterior rami of cervical nerves
Posterior supraclavicular n.
Axillary n.
Intercostobrachial cutaneous
Medial brachial cutaneous n.
Posterior brachial cutaneous (branch of radial n.)
Medial antebrachial cutan. n.
Posterior antebrachial cutaneous n.
Lateral antebrachial cutan. (musculocutaneous) n.
Superficial radial n.
Ulnar n.
Median n.
Lateral femoral cutaneous n.
Anterior femoral cutaneous n.
Posterior femoral cutaneous n.
Common peroneal n.
Superficial peroneal n.
Saphenous n.
Sural n.
Lateral plantar n.
Tibial n.
Medial plantar n.
Posterior thoracic rami
Lateral thoracic rami
Posterior lumbar rami
C-2
C-3
C-4
C-5
C-6
C7
8
T-1
T2
T-2
T-3
T-4
T-5
T-6
T-7
T-8
T-9
T-10
T-11
T-12
L-1
L-2
S-3
S-2
S-1
L 5
L 4
ǂ Iliohypogastric (iliac branch)
* Obturator

Figure 16 B.

such distant placement would have a lesser effect than stimuli placed in the same or adjacent segments.

In addition to evidence of the effectiveness of such spinal, medullary and mid-brain mechanisms, it is well known that the cerebral cortex also plays an important role in pain control (70). Such "down-stream" pain modulating impulses are initiated by a variety of stimuli to sensory and associated areas of the cortex. It has thus been a common observation that distracting sensations (music in the dentist's office, intense interest in a game of sports, etc.) have served to mask otherwise painful stimulation. One can add to distraction other cerebral influences such as emotional set, learned pain behavior patterns, belief, positive thinking, stoicism, etc. It is probable that no one mechanism of pain modulation works entirely in isolation. Evidence that pain control involves at least three types of neurotransmitter systems—opioid, serotonin and norepinephrine—suggests that in any single instance of pain control one or a combination of all three might be involved. The demonstration that hypnotic analgesia does not act through the same opioid mechanisms as acupuncture, suggests that these two forms of pain control—acupuncture and hypnosis—can be additive and thus when used together bring about a more complete suppression of pain.

Also, undoubtedly, the placebo effect is manifest here. It exists for every other type of therapy. Placebos can be effective analgesics and as has been demonstrated by Levine, *et al.* (27), such placebo-induced analgesia is mediated by endorphins. Hence the placebo also acts by way of neurotransmitter systems to modulate nociceptor inputs. Loeser (71) includes in the placebo category such concepts as "entertainment of the patients, fascination with exotic therapies, the desire to please the therapist and the legitimization of an illness when the traditional health care system has failed to clarify a diagnosis or implement successful therapy" He reiterates the well known fact that placebo effect can occur with any form of therapy. If, indeed, some of the above factors are maximized when a patient comes for acupuncture it would seem that here the placebo effect could well be a strong one. Just as "gate control" implies activation of dorsal horn modulating neural mechanisms so "placebo effect" implies activation of cerebral modulating neural mechanisms.

Acupuncture can then, as we have already pointed out, modify the threshold for direction of a noxious stimulus at the point of its entry into the spinal cord, or through ascending mechanisms it can effect analgesia by activating midbrain mechanisms and, in addition, through its placebo effect modulate pain by means of descending cerebral impulses and the recruitment of additional neurotransmitter mechanisms. The fact that acupuncture has a strong "placebo" effect should not deprecate its value for pain relief. The patient is concerned only with obtaining relief from suffering. How the therapeutic manipulation works is, to the patient, of secondary concern. If acupuncture works by both physiologic (neurochemical-physiological) and placebo (psychological-neurochemical) means then it may be stronger by such augmentation than either mechanism alone.

Most chemo-analgesic methods have unwanted side effects of which acupuncture has relatively few. Most chemo-analgesics are extremely time limited and must be repeated usually every few hours of each day. While acupuncture has been criticized for (72), "losing its effectiveness after four months," it should be pointed out that patients who have had many years or months of suffering may, indeed, welcome a simple non-harmful procedure given by means of a relatively few treatments from which they may receive even a limited "four months" of freedom from pain and disagreeable chemo-therapy. In our clinical experience we have had a number of patients followed over a 5-10 year period who have, after years of suffering, experienced complete relief from a short series of electro-acupuncture treatments. This relief lasted over several years duration with the pain then returning only to be again banished but this time by an even shorter series of treatments. There are, of course, many patients who gain only brief respite or whose pain remains unchanged after 8-10 acupuncture treatments. Why the neurotransmitter mechanism should be so readily effected by electro-acupuncture stimulation in one person and not in another remains to be determined. Perhaps with some standardization of technique and careful recording and study of stimulus parameters over many treatments, sufficient knowledge will be gained so that we may expand our success with this technique to include a larger number of patients. Such will be the gain from a scientifically based method of acupuncture.

In our limited experience, transcutaneous electrical nerve stimulation (TENS), with surface electrodes has effected relief only while the current is turned on. Its effect is more like that of an orally administered analgesic in that it is time-limited. Some of our patients have used this apparatus to obtain temporary relief between our once weekly acupuncture treatments. They have then discarded it once acupuncture has brought about permanent relief. Also, TENS stimulation is not without its dangers in that patients can inflict upon themselves serious burns if they are exposed to the stimulus for too long a period of time as when falling asleep with the stimulator turned on.

Further evidence that acupuncture and TENS may work by different mechanisms is found in reports by Zhang (73) and Sjolund (74). These reports, taken together indicate that acupuncture-like stimulation can increase endorphin release in the perfusate of the peri-aqueductual gray, caudate and accumbuns nuclei and that such increased enkephalin concentration in the cerebrospinal fluid does not occur after high frequency transcutaneous nerve stimulation.

Clinically, we are primarily concerned with the long term treatment of pain. The mechanisms described here, which have been elucidated to explain the short term relief of pain by acupuncture may well serve as the basis from which the discovery of the control of chronic pain can be developed. In this regard, it should be mentioned that Wancura and Konig (75), discussed some of these mechanisms in 1974 while much of the work on the opioid neurotransmitter was still in the stage of early investigation. One point they made is worth repeating here, i.e., that the areas in which the most important points for acupuncture are situated correspond to particularly large areas in the sensory homunculus in the thalamus. These areas consist of the trigeminus, the arms and the legs. The representation of a separate zone for the trigeminus region in the sensory homunculus at the base of the thalamus might somehow be related to the fact that about three-fourths of all points required for analgesia are situated in the trigeminal area—in the ear, on the nose and on the face. The most important analgesic points in body acupuncture are situated on the arms and legs, zones that are represented by large areas in both the sensory thalamic homunculus (Figure 17) and, as well, in the post-central sensory area of the cerebral cortex. The thumb has a particularly large representation on the cortex and, among all acupuncture points of the upper limb, ho-ku, (LI-4), is probably the best known and the most frequently utilized. The importance of the sensory cortex in the pain modulation response to acupuncture was shown by the work of Ha and Tan who found that the analgesic effect, induced by stimulation of LI-4 on the left hand is abolished following unilateral ablation of the hand area of the right post-central gyrus (76). As we hypothesize and as Wancura and Konig (75), also mentioned, bathyesthesia or vibration can modify nociception. Thus, stimulation of some or all motor afferents that are carried in the sensory nerves are of great importance for eliciting pain modifying responses. For such reason points on the extremity where there are many muscles and many motor points should be of the greatest importance. Acupuncture theory has long stressed the importance of "ting" points which are on the hands and feet. Ryadorako (77), a form of Japanese acupuncture, makes the greatest use of wrist and ankle points. In our

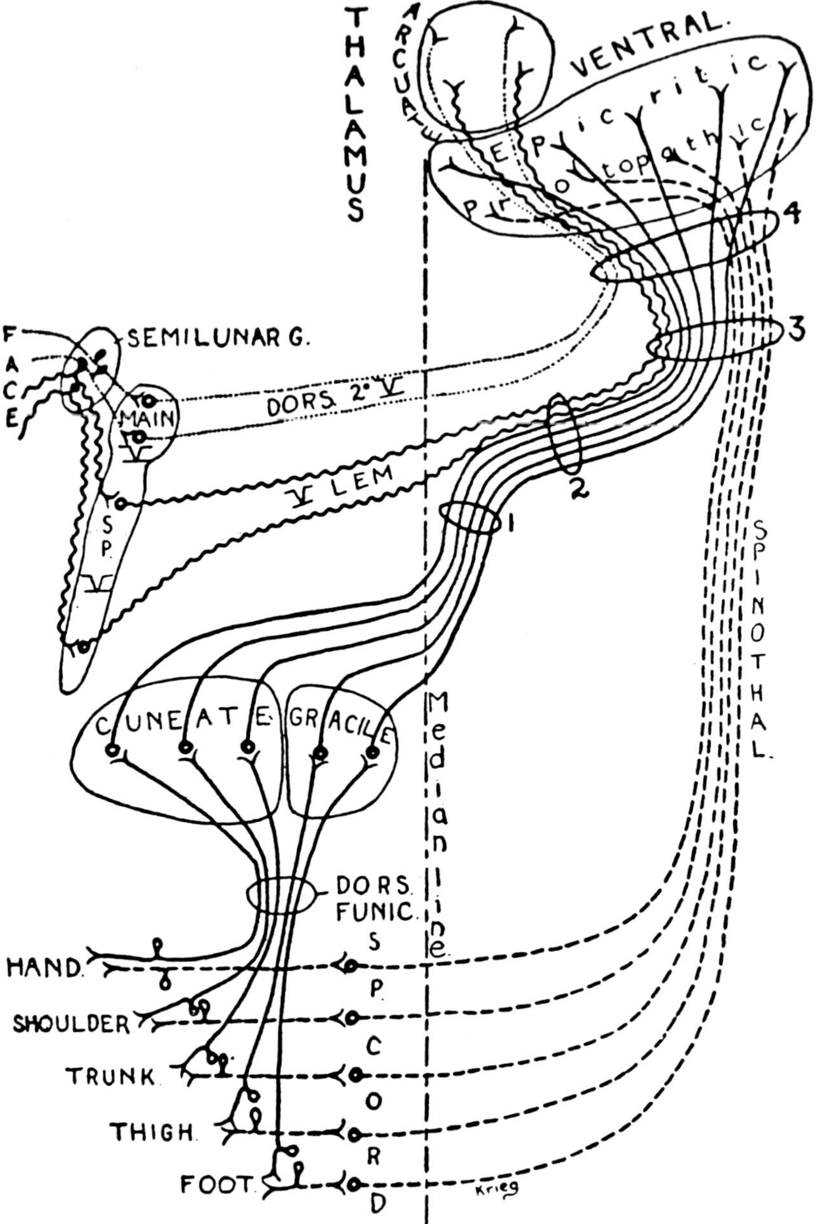

Figure 17. (A) Course of sensory pathways to thalamus. From Krieg, Wendell J.S.: *Functional Neuroanatomy.* McGraw Hill Book Company, New York, Second Edition, 1953. (B) Schematic of thalamic nuclei showing sensory zones.

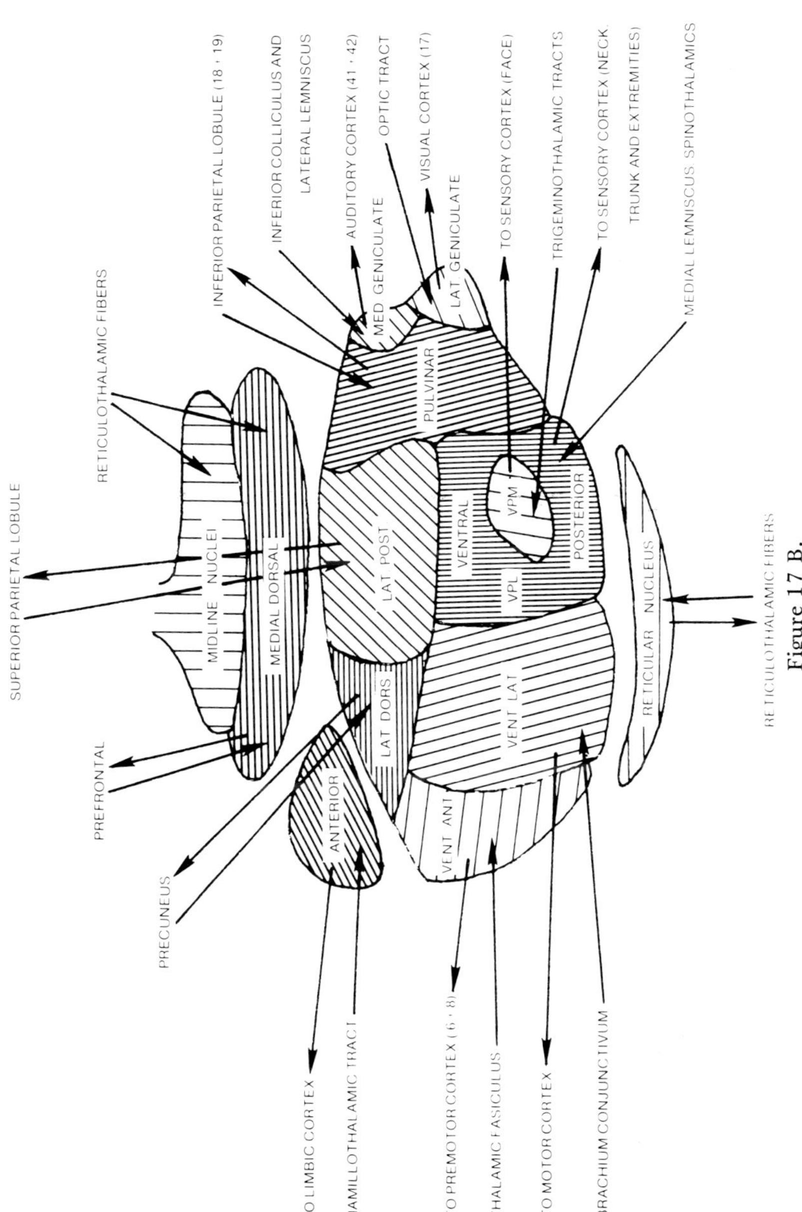
SUPERIOR PARIETAL LOBULE
RETICULOTHALAMIC FIBERS
INFERIOR PARIETAL LOBULE (18, 19)
INFERIOR COLLICULUS AND
LATERAL LEMNISCUS
AUDITORY CORTEX (41, 42)
OPTIC TRACT
VISUAL CORTEX (17)
LAT. GENICULATE
TO SENSORY CORTEX (FACE)
TRIGEMINOTHALAMIC TRACTS
TO SENSORY CORTEX (NECK,
TRUNK AND EXTREMITIES)
MEDIAL LEMNISCUS, SPINOTHALAMICS
MED GENICULATE
PULVINAR
VPM
VENTRAL
POSTERIOR
VPL
LAT. POST
MIDLINE NUCLEI
MEDIAL DORSAL
LAT DORS
VENT LAT
ANTERIOR
VENT ANT
RETICULAR NUCLEUS
RETICULOTHALAMIC FIBERS
PREFRONTAL
PRECUNEUS
TO LIMBIC CORTEX
MAMILLOTHALAMIC TRACT
TO PREMOTOR CORTEX (6, 8)
THALAMIC FASICULUS
TO MOTOR CORTEX
BRACHIUM CONJUNCTIVUM

Figure 17 B.

own research work we found that as one moves down the extremities from proximal to distal it takes less electricity to produce a sensation of the same intensity.

Although the above theories give insight into mechanisms explanatory for the production of analgesia for brief periods of time we must also have some rationale for longer term effects. When acupuncture is used as an analgesic for surgery, stimulation is started 20-40 minutes prior to the operation to permit a build up (recruiting, deepening) of sufficient analgesia to permit surgery with sensation but without pain. When the analgesia-producing electro-acupuncture stimulation is stopped, it has been observed that, while diminishing, the effect lasts over a period of 30 minutes or more. What then might be the mechanism for relief from chronic pain over longer periods of time and even permanently?

It seems probable on the basis of known physiology that, in establishing conditions of chronic pain, the ancient, slowly conducting system of C-fibers takes dominion over the more phylogenetically recent, rapidly conducting myelinated fibers. With continuing stimulation from tissue damage or irritation, the pain becomes continuous or chronically intermittently occuring. Such continuous bombardment of the neuraxis by noxious stimuli could well produce a kindling (78) within neurone pools of the central nervous system such that reverberating circuits are created with self-perpetuation or continuation of the pain sensations with mechanisms after the fashion early described by Lorente-de-No (79), Dusser de Baren (80) and others (Figure 18). Such circuits at the spinal cord level have been described in the de-afferented spinal cord in a patient with continuing paraplegic pain, by Loesser, Ward and White (81). This self-generated abnormal bursting activity in the spinal cord has also been described by the above workers in the cat with chronic deafferentation.

Such spinal reverberating circuits could serve to constantly activate midbrain and cortical circuits via ascending pathways. This might explain the continuing memory of pain in the central nervous system long after the original tissue injury has been repaired. In the case of phantom limb pain, it would appear that the activity continues to reverberate in the central circuits previously utilized by the now non-existent limb.

An alternative mechanism may be related to a malfunction of the system for production and control of brain hormones that relate to the pain experience (Figure 19). Thus, the noxious impulses could well produce a dysregulation of those homeostatic mechanisms that are responsible for a return to the resting stage after a warning for the location and extent of tissue damage has been given. A continuing or very intense

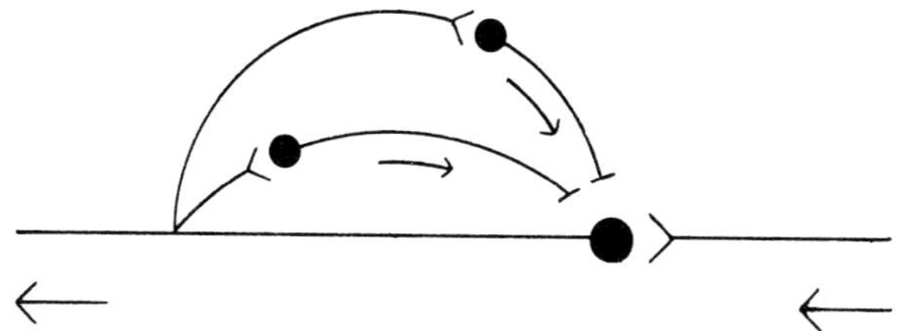

Figure 18. Schematic of reverberating neurone circuits in the central nervous system.

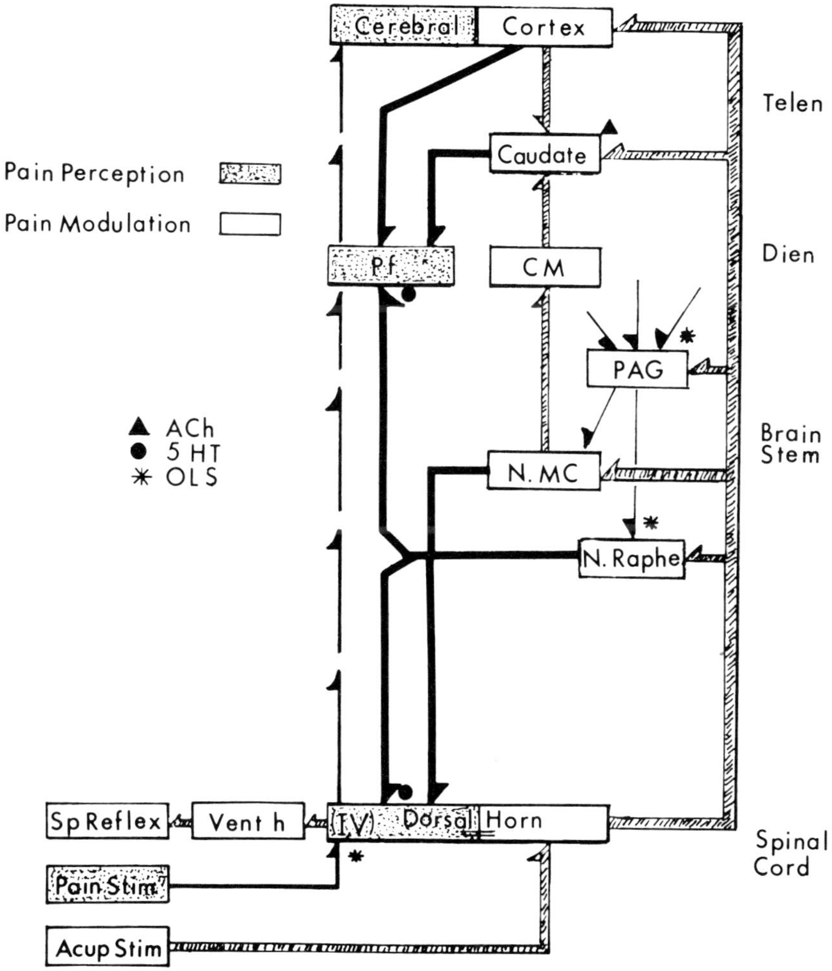

Figure 19. Schematic of brain hormone systems that modulate pain mechanisms in the central nervous system. From Han, C.S., Tang, J., Jen, M.F., Zhou, A.F., Fan, S.G., and Qio, X.C.: The role of central neurotransmitters in acupuncture analgesia. Private Publication. *Research Group of Acupuncture Anesthesia.* Peking, People's Republic of China.

pain stimulus could, presumably result in either an excessive production of the peptides responsible for the transmission of pain impulses or a breakdown in the function of those structures responsible for the production of enkephalins necessary for suppression of neuronal activity in the pain pathways.

When the pain impulse spreads to involve the intermediolateral column of the spinal cord the sympathetic nervous system is activated (Figure 20) and its dysregulation results in causalgia (82). Here the cardinal signs are burning pain, trophic changes (glossy skin) and often a local rise in temperature. If left untreated hyperalgesia occurs, muscles become fibrosed, osteoporosis may occur and often there is accompanying emotional lability.

Other post-traumatic pain syndromes as described by Livingston (82), include a peculiar distribution of pain. He describes a "mirror image" pain in which pain develops in the non-involved side at the precise mirrored location of the contralateral lesion. Such phenomena are explained by the spread of uncontrolled pain by neurons crossing the midline or by spread of excitation by neurohumors to involve other neuron galaxies in the spinal cord within the same segment but on the opposite side. He has also emphasized the importance of recognizing neurotome distribution, which we feel is an important principle in acupuncture treatment. An example is his "multifidus triangle syndrome". Here the innervation of the multifidus muscle by S1,S2,S3 may refer pain both in the lateral thigh and the sciatic distribution in the lower leg.

Livingston points out that, "In many of the causalgic states which have been long established, the higher centers become affected and all manner of physiologic and even organic changes may take place in parts of the body far removed from the original focus of irritation." In many clinical syndromes there may be a combination of somatic, visceral and psychic irritation each contributing to the central process. Once a vicious cycle is established the process tends to become self-sustaining. In our experience it usually takes repeated acupuncture sessions to break up such long standing pain mechanisms.

The very complexity of the pain phenomenon makes it likely that several different mechanisms are at work and that pain relief, even from a single treatment measure like acupuncture, may be accomplished by several different mechanisms. Gunn (22), in a series of papers, has, without negating the importance of the gate theory, suggested yet another mechanism by which needle therapy may work. He points out that pain is not a sensation in the strict neurophysiologic sense because there is no direct relation between the intensity of the applied stimulus

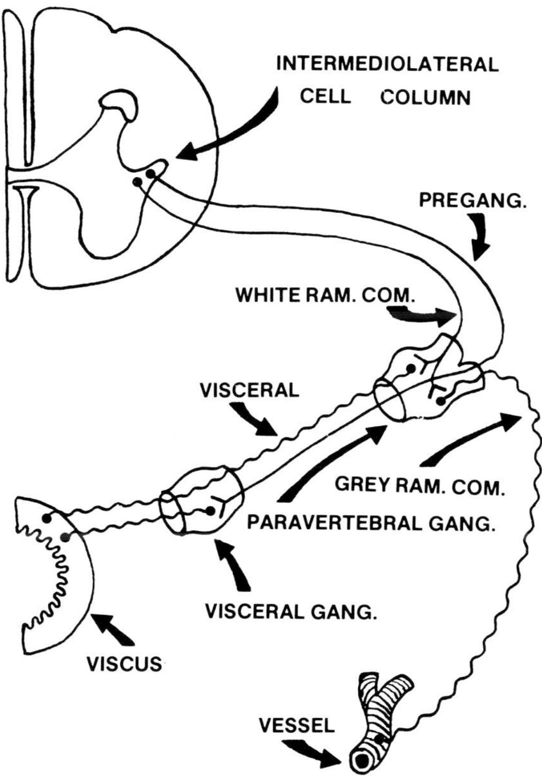

Figure 20. Relationship of the sympathetic nervous system to the intermediolateral cell column of the spinal cord.

and the impulse discharge frequency or between the stimulus and the intensity of the pain experience. He points out that myofascial pain is often the result of spondylosis, that as a part of the aging process, degenerative changes occur in the intervertebral disc with narrowing of the intervertebral foramina (Figure 21). Two types of degeneration then occur, either axonal neuropathy or segemental demyelinization. Both usually occur with varying degrees of damage and reversibility. In accord with Cannon's Law of Denervation, the muscle and peripheral receptors become hypersensitive to transmitter substances and to various forms of stimuli. In normal muscle, acetycholine receptor sites are confined to the region of the end plates. After denervation, the area sensitive to acetylcholine spreads along the surface membrane of the entire fiber. As segmental nerves are of a mixed character, changes can occur in both afferent and efferent fibers, thus affecting motor, sensory and autonomic functions. Location of pain from such root located disturbance may be in the corresponding myotome, (muscle pain and tenderness), dermatome (numbness, deadness or tingling), or in the sclerotome (dull aching, burning pain, deep and difficult to localize), or in the autonomic fibers producing prolonged burning pain and the vasomotor changes of sympathetic reflex dystrophy (causalgia). The tender motor points that develop from such root injury produce a variety of clinical pictures and often lead to misdiagnoses of bursitis, rotator cuff syndrome, etc.

According to Gunn's theory, treatment with needle puncture at the motor point (neurovascular hilus) produces locally a current of injury that persists over several days until the micro-wound heals. With successive treatment multiple microtraumata occur with the formation of scar tissue which ultimately displaces a number of functioning nociceptors and, thus, gives prolonged or permanent relief from chronic pain. Also, the needles produce analgesia by stimulation of the larger diameter myelinated fibers found at the motor point in accordance with the mechanism of the gate theory. Such current injury has been shown experimentally to reduce the denervation hypersensitivity to acetylcholine.

As can be seen from the foregoing discussion, there is not one simple explanation of how acupuncture works. Rather, there are a number of plausible mechanisms several or all which may be effective simultaneously. There is no one theory to explain the effectiveness of acupuncture treatment. There are however several theories, backed by considerable factual knowledge, to explain some of its effectiveness, particularly that part which is concerned with the control of acute pain, both somatic and visceral.

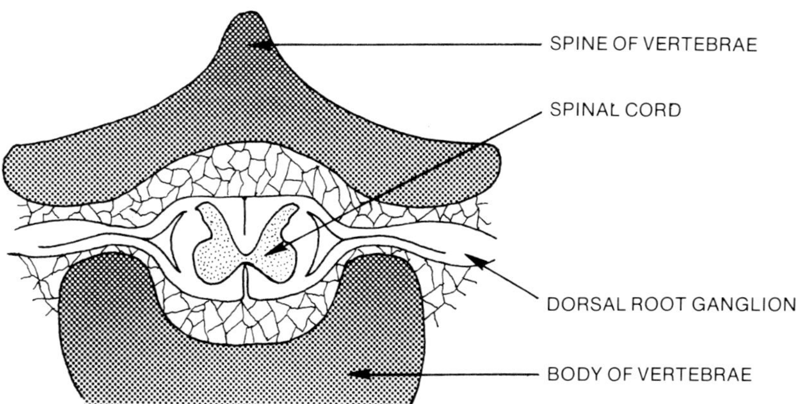

Figure 21. Exit of spinal nerves from the intervertebral foraminae.

Acupuncture has been reported to be of assistance in the promotion of healing. It is known that nuclei of the median reticular formation have intimate connections with the hypothalamus and, hence, could affect vegetative homeostatic regulatory mechanisms. Indeed, this may be the anatomical substrate for the effects upon blood pressure, pulse, respiration, intestinal motility, increase in white blood cells and hormone secretion that have been described to occur with acupuncture (83,84).

Another important mechanism could be direct reflex stimulation via the pathways for cutaneo-visceral reflexes within the same neurotome segments whereby visceral and somato-motor innervation lie within identical or adjacent segments. Such mechanisms are well known and have been described by McKenzie (85), Kellgren (86) and Head (87). Yet another aid to healing can occur simply from the muscle relaxation that results following the relief of pain for it is well known that increased tonus and spasm of muscle is a common accompaniment of pain and that it can interfere with adequate blood supply and nutrition to damaged tissue. Pain relief through acupuncture can relieve such spasm and thus improve tissue healing.

Acupuncture has been widely reported to be effective in conditions other than pain and such claims are found throughout the literature on traditional Chinese medicine. Reports suggesting that acupuncture may influence the cardiovascular system have been published by Omura (83), Tam (88) and others. Thus, as has been pointed out by Liao (89), acupuncture needle stimulation of cutaneous and muscle nerves in neurotome areas can produce a direct and immediate effect on sympathetic nerve activities.

Andersson and his collaborators (84), have reported from studies using spontaneously hypertensive rats, that acupuncture-like stimulation of the sciatic nerve at a frequency of three Hz and an intensity sufficient to activate A-delta fibers produced an initial elevation in blood pressure and heart rate and decreased splanchnic nerve activity. This reaction, from 30 minutes of stimulation, reached a peak in one hour and produced depressive effects lasting up to twelve hours. This effect is naloxone reversible suggesting involvement of the endorphin system known also to be the mediator of the hyperalgesia seen with sciatic nerve stimulation.

These workers also found evidence of involvement of the central serotonin system which too has been shown to be concerned with the modulation of blood pressure by changing the level of sympathetic activity (84). This latter may be mediated by the acupuncture effect to increase B-endorphin secretion together with ACTH from the pituitary. It is evident that there is an inter-relationship between the endorphin and the serotonin systems in the regulation of the cardiovascular as well as the nociceptive systems.

We have puzzled long over auriculotherapy and feel that here, as with much of traditional acupuncture, a single grain of truth from empiric observation has been greatly expanded by an overly enthusiastic interpretation of clinical results abetted by a lack of controlled observations. Without doubt, however, the innervation of the concha of the ear by the vagus nerve is an anatomical fact of considerable importance. The vagus nucleus lies in the midst of the reticular pathways of the brain stem beset by numerous interconnections. There is no research validation of the widely described topical relationships of individual points on the ear to discrete body areas. It does however appear logical that stimulation anywhere in the concha (the vagus nerve area of the ear) could well activate parasympathetic mechanisms reaching widely throughout the body. Such activation can result in modification of visceral functions by stimulating a vagal discharge. This, in turn, would modulate the activity in all of the viscera supplied by this parasympathetic regulating mechanism. As an antidote for excess sympathetic stimulation which produces both anxiety and organ hyperactivity such stimulation of the ear area innervated by the vagus nerve could well act to restore homeostatic balance. We have found clinically that such stimulation can produce a marked anti-anxiety and relaxing effect.

Mendelson (90), points to similarities between alcohol and narcotic withdrawal syndromes with their preponderance of excessive sympathetic (adrenergic) activity. He presents evidence that such symptoms are suppressed both by cholingeric agents and, as well, by ear electro-acupuncture. This gives support to our own contention that stimulation of the concha of the ear is a useful technique for the relief of anxiety in psychiatric patients in whom such excessive sympathetic overactivity is a prominent symptom. This effective suppression of sympathetic hyperactivity by vagal (parasympathetic) activation may be the sole foundation upon which the otherwise elaborate and unsupported structure of auriculotherapy has been built.

Psychiatrists have long been concerned with the pain/pleasure dipole (91), which refers to extremes in the mechanism of psychic homeostasis. The work of Old's (92), demonstrated the existence of pleasure centers in the brain. Sleep researchers have described a system in the midbrain that controls the sleep-wakefulness cycle and presents a neuro-chemical basis for reducing vigilance (93) and promoting a mental state (sleep) that eliminates both pain and dysphoria. L-tryptophan, the serotonin precursor, has been shown to be useful in promoting sleep and also elevating pain threshold (94). Thus, both anatomically and neurohumorally, areas for pleasure, sleep, and the relief of pain may be related.

Thus, in conclusion, there are a host of mechanisms, some well-documented, others less well and some as yet quite theoretical, but all scientifically possible, by which acupuncture could exert an effect for calming, comfort and the relief of pain in patients who are plagued by chronic suffering and depression.

As this book goes to press we have become aware of a recent publication of Han and Terenius.* Their article presents an extensive review of the literature on the neurochemical basis of acupuncture. It includes reports not easily accessible to the general scientific community. Much important work has been done by the two authors. This article warrants the serious attention of all physicians.

*Han, J.S., and Terenius, L.: Neurochemical basis of acupuncture analgesia. *Ann. Rev. Pharmacol. Toxicol.*, 1982, 22:193-220.

V

NEEDLING POINTS AND TREATMENT STRATEGIES

By tradition, there are some 360 acupuncture points. Over the centuries, practitioners, for whatever reasons, added other points. The expansion of auriculotheraphy, the advent of acupuncture "anesthesia" and the recent rebirth of interest in acupuncture throughout the world have, altogether, resulted in an increase of points used over the body until the number described to-date reaches 1,000. The ancient Chinese taught that the acupuncture points served as holes on the meridians where the passage of energy might be affected. These points were located along hypothetical lines known as meridians with their exact identification dependent upon local landmarks of the body such as body tubercules, nipples, depressions in muscular structure and the like. Once the approximate location of the point had been determined it was stated that careful palpation could reveal a slight depression in the subcutaneous tissue. Some points were said to be tender to pressure, others were felt as nodules. These meridians of traditional acupuncture are purely a hypothetical taxonomic concept and have nothing to do with the forces of energy or physiology.

Useful acupunture may be practiced with knowledge of the location of some 50-75 physiologically active points. As will be explained in this chapter most of such useful points coincide with motor points and lie close to nerve trunks or Golgi tendon organs. In principle, points for effective stimulation lie within the domain of the neurotome corresponding to the area of disturbance and as such are capable of evoking changes in visceral as well as somatic tissues. Those points that are tender or nodular-like are often trigger points.

Originally such physiologically active points as described above were discovered serendipidously. They became enshrouded in the meridian theory and soon lost among dozens of other lesser or inactive points that became incorporated into traditional acupuncture theory over the centuries. It has only been recently that the more active acupuncture points were found to coincide with known motor point or nerve trunk locations.

Our own work (95), has demonstrated that many of these points have a strong electrical potential, positive or negative and up to 42 millivolts. Such electrical identity has led to the development of electrical point locators that operate on the basis of lowered skin resistance. These instruments utilize a roving electrode and a ground electrode and permit the passage of a small electrical current to measure local changes in skin resistance. Either a movement of the indicator on a meter or a change in sound from a small speaker demonstrates the different resistance of an active point. Repeated measurement, changes in pressure of the electrodes, sweating, etc., can cause false measurement and, hence, this system of point location is frought with considerable error. Such instruments are, therefore, without any practical clinical value.

The basic principle of point selection for needle placement may be most simply expressed as locating an area of the body where stimulation will produce a beneficial change in the central nervous system through a modulation of ongoing activity. Such points usually lie within or near the neural segment that supplies innervation to the afflicted area. Needle placement should, therefore, be in a motor point, adjacent to a major afferent nerve, within a neural plexus, at a trigger point or at a point of somato-visceral reference. In this way the stimulation permits access to that part of the neuraxis where the noxious disturbance has its origin. Such areas will ordinarly lie within the neurotome (dermatome or myotome) of the troubled area.

The hypothesized events that occur following stimulation of such points begin first at the point of entry of the stimulus into the central nervous system. This is, at the spinal cord level, presumably in the substantia gelatinosa where the entering impulses from afferent nerve stimulation of A-delta fibers block the more slowly traveling impulses of nocicpetive fibers. Secondly, following such events, impulses ascend to similar gating mechanisms at higher levels in the central nervous system and produce even longer lasting influences upon the neurochemistry of the brain through increasing the production and liberation of pain relieving neuro-transmitting substances including the endorphins. With repeated stimulation there is an interruption and ultimately dissolution of reverberating circuits whose self-repetitive nature is undoubtedly the basis for a continuation of the original pathological pain stimulus. Thus, it is our belief from our own observations and the experiences of Mann (98), Gunn (22) and others that, in the main, points for treatment may be usefully selected on the basis of such neuro-anatomical and neurophysiological principles. We will explore the selection of such areas for stimulation in greater detail. We will also present some of the formulae for multiple needle placement that have been handed down through the centuries as points that have been found useful for specific afflictions, emphasizing wherever possible those points which, although originally selected empirically, seem to have some rationale in modern scientific terms. In the main we will stress that the selection of acupuncture points for the treatment of any condition should be based upon producing a stimulus in those areas of the central nervous system which refer to the region of pain or disturbance. Such selection will, therefore, rely primarily upon a knowledge of neurotome distribution rather than any dependence upon traditional acupuncture theory for the location of meridian points. As Felix Mann wisely pointed out (98), once such neurophysiological principles are understood, a Western doctor may practice scientific acupuncture while "the ancients had good results by acupuncture (but) for the wrong reasons."

In addition to the selection of points on a regional basis depending upon the area of pain or dysfunction, there seems to be a general effect operating regardless of where the needle is placed. Thus, many patients report an overall feeling of relaxation or improvement which could be explained in terms of some of the humoral theories of acupuncture mechanism which have been described (99,100,101).

A. SELECTION OF MOTOR POINTS FOR STIMULATION

Recent studies that have compared acupuncture points with motor points (the neurovascular hilus points of electromyography) have found precise concordance in at least 35 points (96,97). Many other acupuncture points are located close enough to motor points so that electrical stimulation can activate the motor point even when such a point is not in an exactly concordant location. Gunn (22), described other useful acupuncture points as those located at a focal meeting of superficial nerves in the anterior saggital plane. Other useful points lie over nerve trunks or nerve plexuses. Table II and the accompanying figures ((22-a-x), list the points that we have found useful in our clinical practice. The majority of these are motor points or lie close to the areas where motor points are likely to be found. Thus in many of the figures we have shown the more traditional acupuncture point and in an adjacent drawing motor points located nearby. We use these points interchangeably for, with electrical stimulation, if the needle is located with only approximate accuracy it simply requires a boost in current to produce an appreciation of the stimulus sensation. A rhythmic pulsation of the needle indicates that efferent motor (muscle) stimulation has been achieved as well as afferent sensory involvement.

TABLE II

SEVENTY-FIVE USEFUL POINTS FOR ACUPUNCTURE TREATMENT

HEAD

REGION	NAME	ANATOMICAL LOCATION	PHYSIOLOGIC JUSTIFICATION
Vertex	GV-20	Bisection of sagittal line with line joining tragi	Supraorbital n. meets C_2 C_3
Temporal	EM-1	At midpoint of a line one finger-breath to lateral end of eyebrow and outer canthus of eye	Auriculo temporal n. Deep temporal br. of V n.
Supra-Orbital	BL-2	Above supraorbital notch	Corrugator motor point. Supraorbital br. of V n. Temporal and infra-orbital n. of VII n.
Mid-Infra-Orbital	ST-1	Just above inferior orbital region	Orbicularis oculi motor point. Infra-orbital br. of V n. Facial n.
Median Canthus	BL-1	Just above median canthus	Infratrochlear n. of V
Inferior Masseter	ST-6	Junction of upper 2/3 to lower 1/3 of masseter	Masseter motor point of V
Anterior Mastoid	TH-17	Posterior to the lobule of the auricle and in the depression between the mastoid process and the ramus of the mandible	Lesser occipital n. C_2 C_3 Greater auricular n. C_2 C_3
Mandibular	TH-21	With mouth open, tempero-mandibular joint.	Auriculo temporal n. Facial n.
Nasolabial Fold	LI-20	Nasolabial fold within the fold of cheek at level of inferior edge of ala nasi	Infraorbital br. of V. Buccal br. of VII

(Head Cont'd.)

TABLE II (Cont'd.)

REGION	NAME	ANATOMICAL LOCATION	PHYSIOLOGIC JUSTIFICATION
Infra-Nasal	GV-26	Midline in the orbicularis oris, 2/3 superior to the margin of upper lip	Infracrbital br. of V. Zygomatic br. of VII.
Anterior Tragus	SI-19	In front of the tragus at the depression made when the mouth is slightly open	Auriculo temporal br. of V. Facial n.
Lateral Oral Angle	ST-4	1/2 cm lateral to angle of mouth	Orbicularis oris motor point mental n. Cervico facial br. of VII n.
Antero-Lateral Mandible	ST-5	Inferior edge of mandible anterior to the gonion, lower anterior border of masseter muscle	Buccal ramus of facial nerve.
Anterior Ear	ST-7	Under the zygomatic arch in front of the condyle of the mandible. In the hollow that fills upon opening the jaw	Branches of the temporal and internal pterygoid nerves

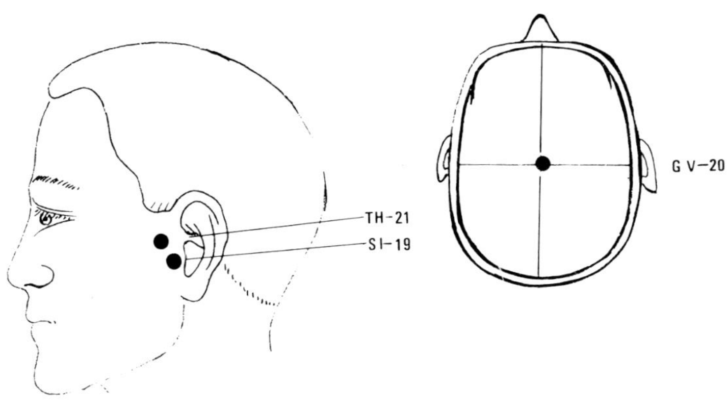

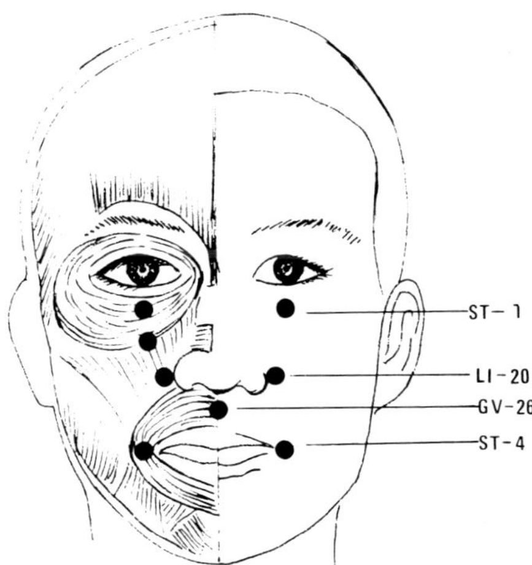

Figure 22. a — x. Seventy five useful acupuncture points with some corresponding or nearby motor points.*
(*After Delagi, E.F., and Perotto, A.: *Anatomic Guide for the Electromyographer*. Charles C. Thomas, Springfield, Ill., 1980.)

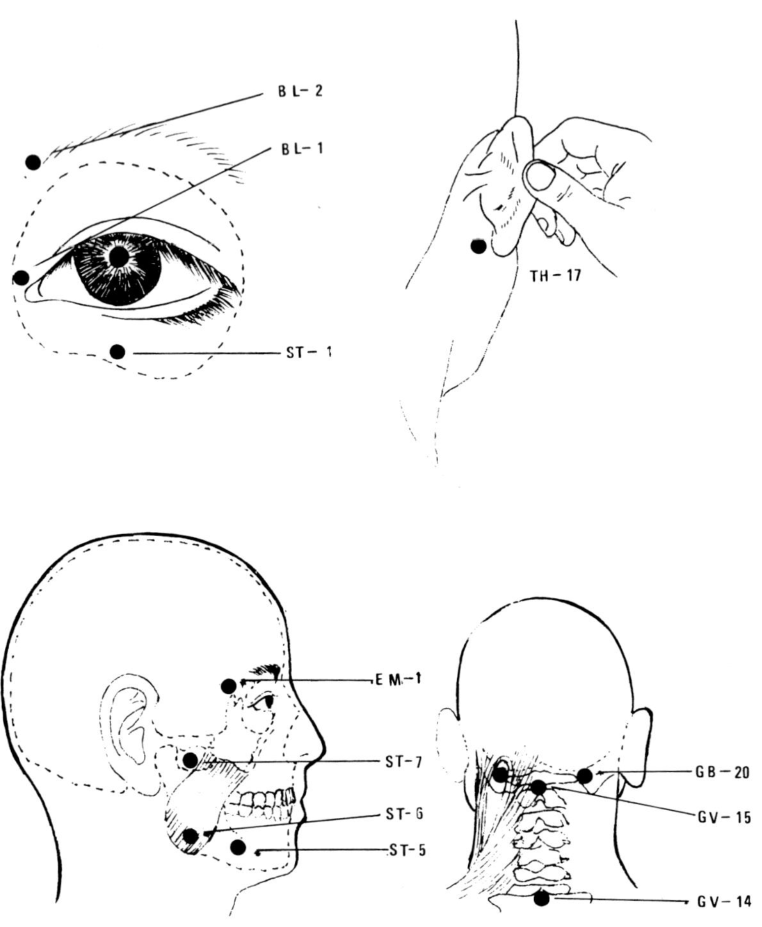

Figure 22 B.

TABLE II (Cont'd.)

NECK

REGION	NAME	ANATOMICAL LOCATION	PHYSIOLOGIC JUSTIFICATION
Sub-occipital	GB-20	Just lateral to trapezius at occiput	Greater occipital C_2 posterior primary ramus
Supraspinous Ligament	GV-15	Supraspinous ligament between C_1-C_2 spinous process midline	Posterior ramus C_2 meets C_3
Paracricoid	ST-9	Anterior border of sterno-mastoid at level of cricoid	Cervical br. of facial n. anterior cutaneous C_2, C_3
Supra-Sternal	CV-22	Neck extended just above sternal notch	Anterior cutaneous n. of neck C_2, C_3
Supra-Spinous Ligament C_7-D_1	GV-14	In the supraspinal ligament, flex head just below C_7 (most prominent spinous process)	Posterior ramus C_3 meets C_4
Sterno-Cleido Mastoid	LI-18	Two fingerbreaths lateral to the mid-point of the laryngeal prominence and between the two heads of the sternocleido-mastoid muscle	Spinal accessory n. (motor) C_2 C_3 (sensory)

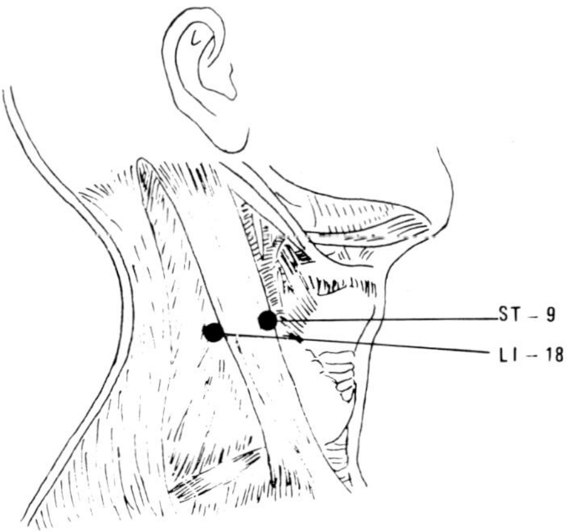

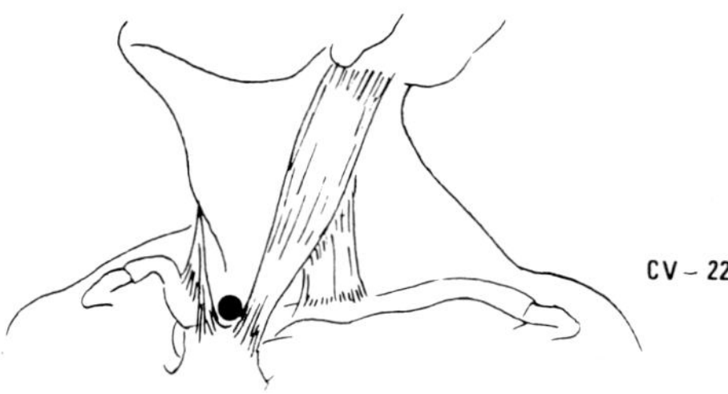

Figure 22 C.

TABLE II (Cont'd.)

CHEST AND ABDOMEN

REGION	NAME	ANATOMICAL LOCATION	PHYSIOLOGICAL JUSTIFICATION
Anterior Shoulder	SP-20	Second intercostal space 8 finger-breaths from midline	Motor point of pectoralis
Upper Lateral Arm	LU-2	Below the acromial extremity of the clavicle in the depression between deltoid and the pectoralis major	Anterior deltoid motor point
Subxiphoid	CV-15	Just below xiphoid process	D_6 and D_7 intercostal anterior cutaneous br. of anterior rami of intercostal
Inframammary	ST-18	Over 5th intercostal space at nipple line	Obliquus externus motor point
Mid-epigas-trium	CV-12	Midpoint between Xiphoid and umbilicus	D_8 and D_9 (bilateral)
Lateral Umbilicus	ST-25	Mid rectus abdominus 2 inch lateral to the umbilicus	Rectus abdominus motor point
Upper Hypogastrium	CV-6	1/5 distance between umbilicus and pubis in midline	Anterior primary ramus (bilateral) D_{11} and D_{12}
Lower Hypogastrium	CV-3	4/5 distance between umbilicus and pubis in midline	Anterior primary ramus (bilateral) D_{12} and L_1 (iliohypogastric)
Suprapubic	CV-2	Just above symphysis pubis	Anterior primary ramus (bilateral) L_1 meets S_2

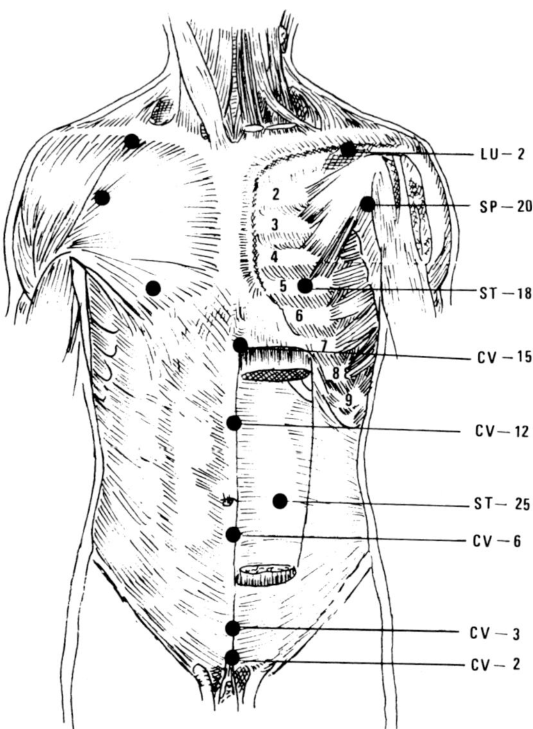

Figure 22 D.

TABLE II (Cont'd.)

UPPER EXTREMITY

REGION	NAME	ANATOMICAL LOCATION	PHYSIOLOGIC JUSTIFICATION
First Dorsal Space	LI-4	1st dorsal interosseious	1st dorsal interosseous motor point
4th Dorsal Space	TH-3	Bet. 4-5 metacarpals	4th dorsal interosseous motor point
5th Lateral Metacarpal	SI-3	Ulnar border of and at distal palmar crease (clenched fist)	Abductor digiti quinti motor point
Dorsal Distal Forearm	TH-5	3 cm proximal to distal end of radius and ulna	Extensor pollicis longus motor point
Dorsal Upper Forearm	TH-9	10 cm distal to olecranon	Extensor carpi ulnaris motor point
Lateral Cubital Crease	LI-11	With elbow flexed, at lateral cubital crease	Brachioradialis motor point
Volar Distal Forearm	PC-6	3 cm proximal to proximal crease over median nerve	Median nerve
Acromio-Clavicula Joint	LI-16	Acromioclavicular joint	Supraclavicular n. (C4)
Posterior Acromion	TH-14	Posterior aspect of acromion	Supraclavicular n. (C_{3-4})

(Upper Extremity Cont'd.)

TABLE II (Cont'd.)

REGION	NAME	ANATOMICAL LOCATION	PHYSIOLOGIC JUSTIFICATION
Posterior Axillary Crease	SI-9	Apex of posterior axillary fold	D_2 D_3 meets circumflex n. C_5 C_6
Posterior Elbow	TH-10	Posterior surface of arm, just above the point of the elbow, junction of triceps muscle with tendon	Muscle tendon junction Golgi tendon organ
Radial Styloid Process	HT-7	Ulnar side of wrist on posterior border of pisiform in depression at radial side of tendon of flexor carpi ulnaris	Medial antebrachial cutaneous n. (T_1); palmar cutaneous branch of the ulnar n. (C_8, T_1); Ulnar n. (C_8, T_1)
Radial Styloid Process	LU-7	Above styloid process of radius, two fingerbreaths above transverse crease of wrist	Lateral antibrachial cutaneous n. ($C_{7,8}$). Superficial branch of the radial n.
Top of Shoulder	GB-21	Top of shoulder in midline between C_7 and acromion	Posterior branch of the supra-clavicular n. and branches of the cervical plexus
Upper Arm	LI-14	Lateral arm at insertion of deltoid	Auxillary n. posterior cord, posterior division upper trunk C_5 C_6

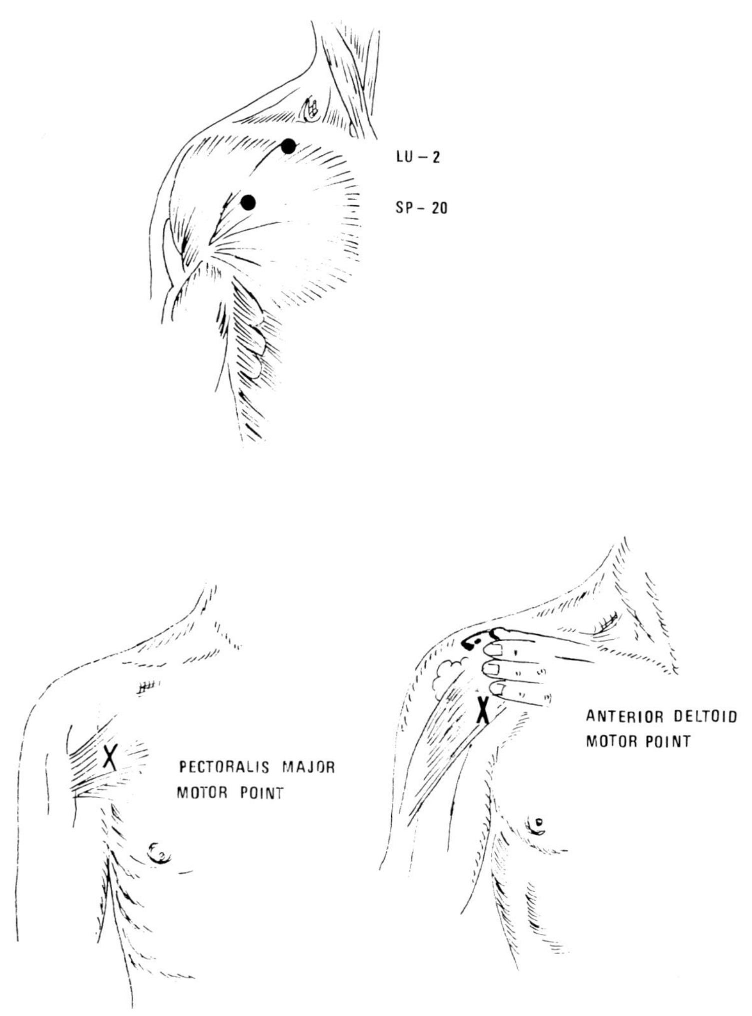
LU – 2
SP – 20
PECTORALIS MAJOR
MOTOR POINT
ANTERIOR DELTOID
MOTOR POINT

Figure 22 E.

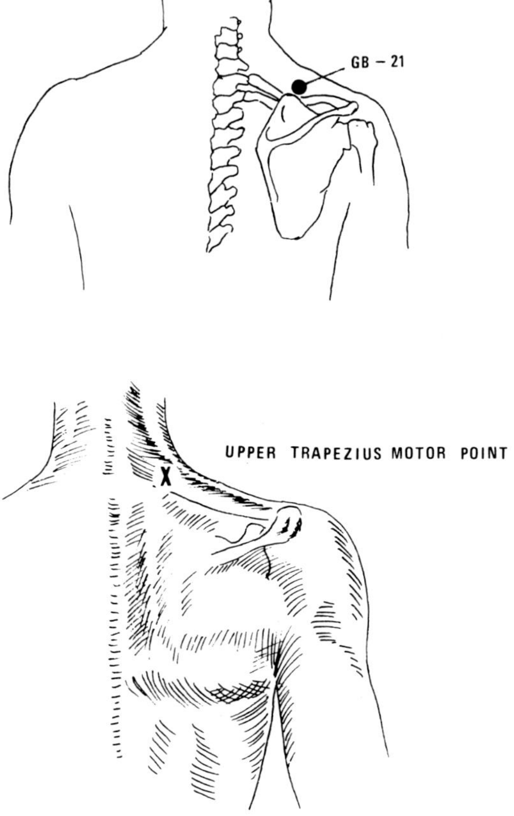

Figure 22 F.

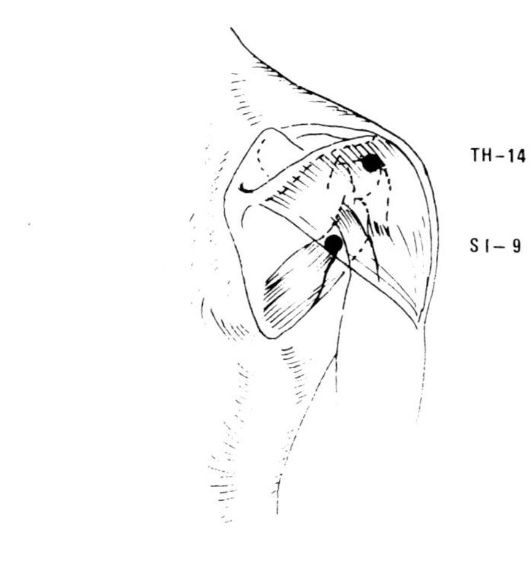

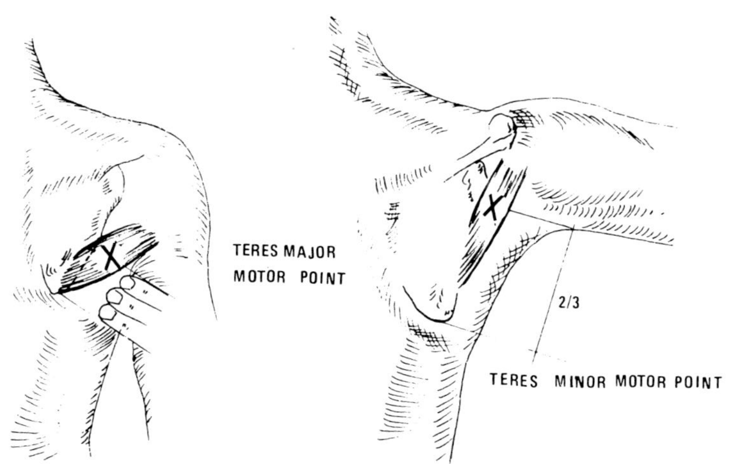

Figure 22 G.

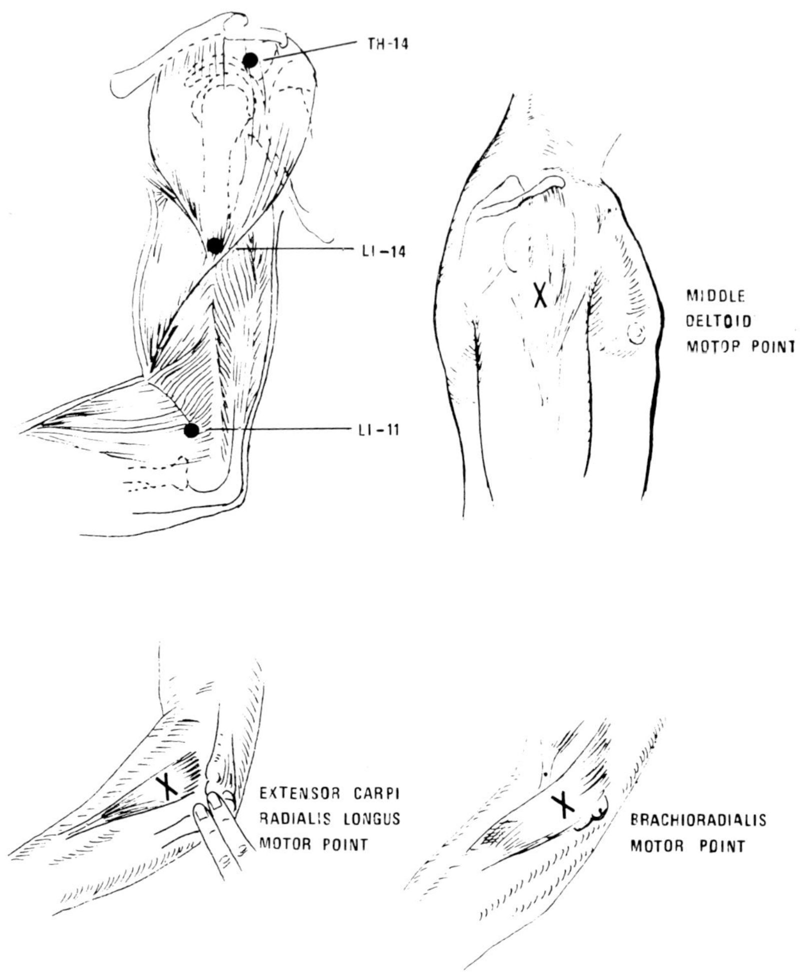
TH-14
LI-14
LI-11
MIDDLE
DELTOID
MOTOP POINT
EXTENSOR CARPI
RADIALIS LONGUS
MOTOR POINT
BRACHIORADIALIS
MOTOR POINT

Figure 22 H.

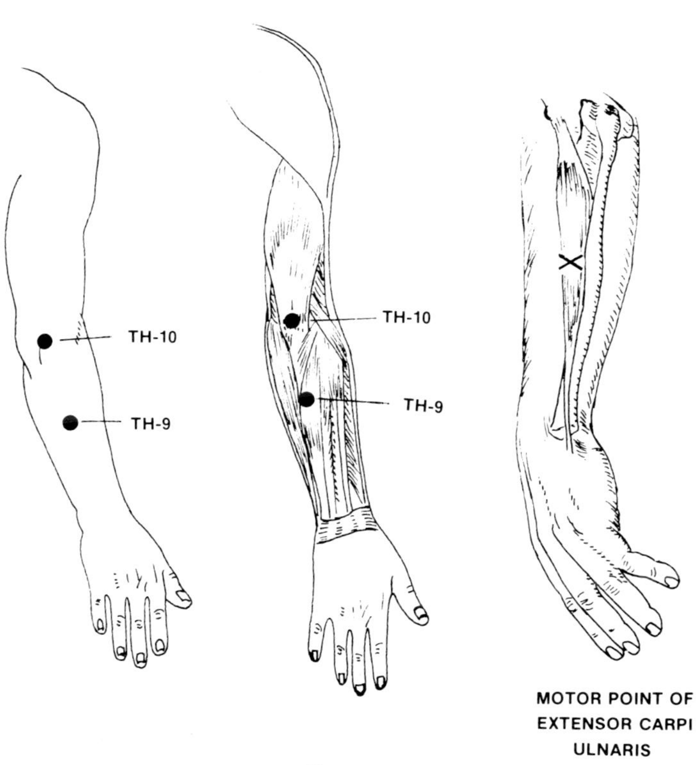

Figure 22 I.

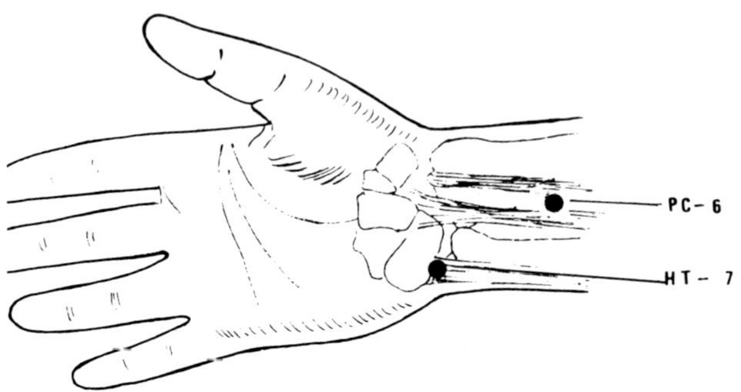

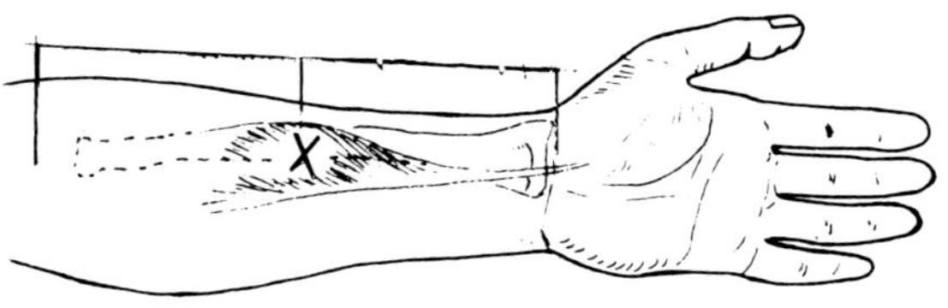

FLEXOR POLLICIS LONGUS MOTOR POINT

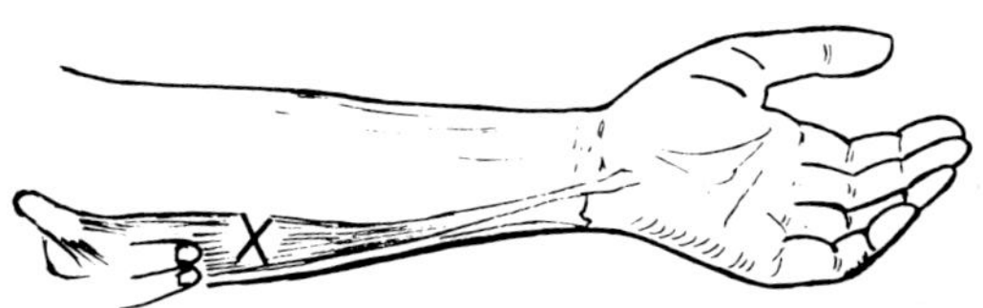

FLEXOR CARPI ULNARIS MOTOR POINT

Figure 22 J.

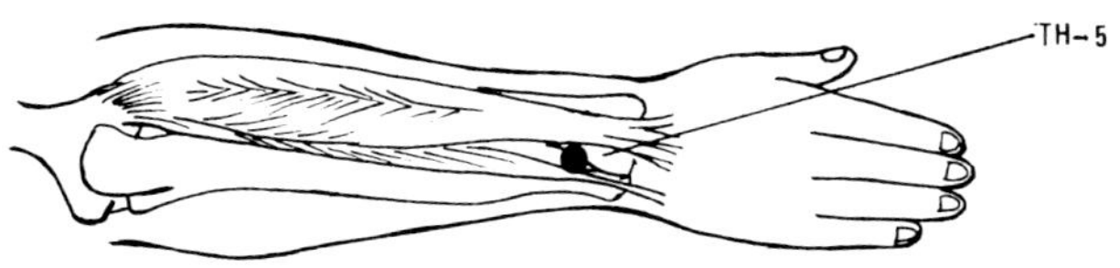

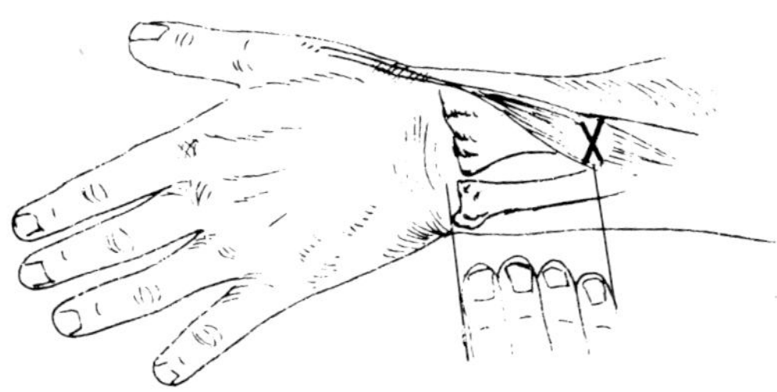

EXTENSOR POLLICIS BREVIS MOTOR POINT

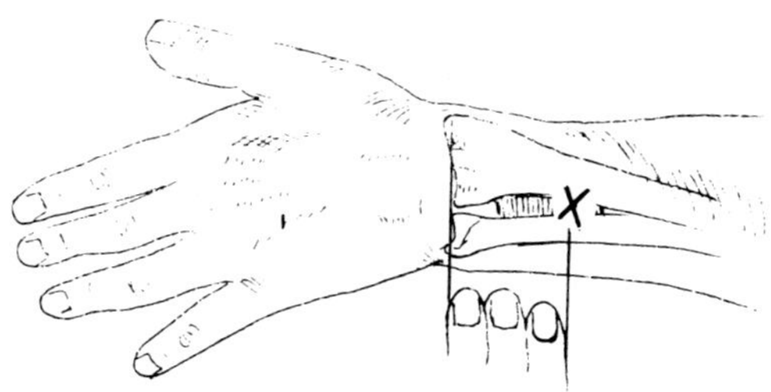

PRONATOR QUADRATUS MOTOR POINT

Figure 22 K.

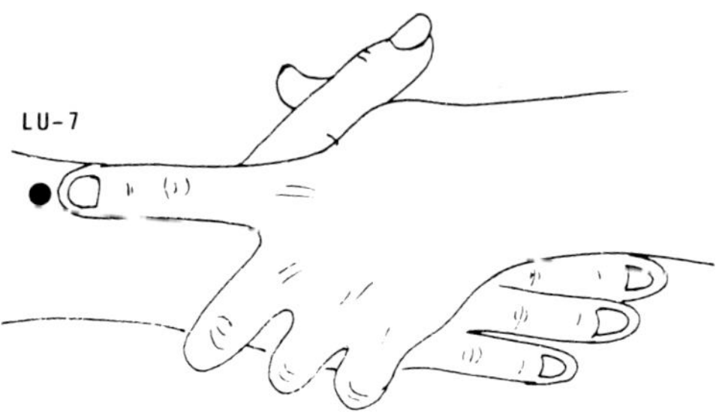

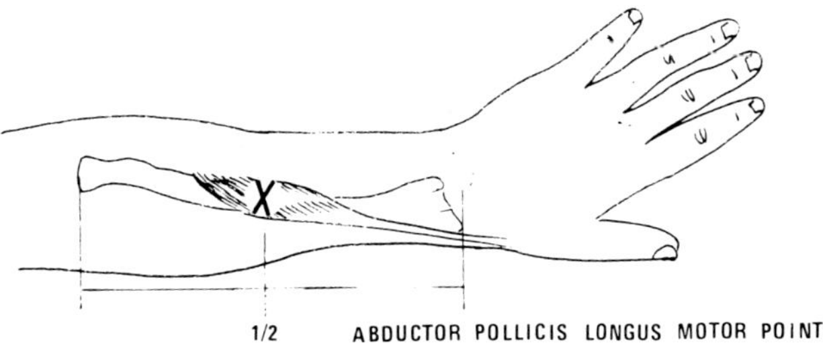

Figure 22 L.

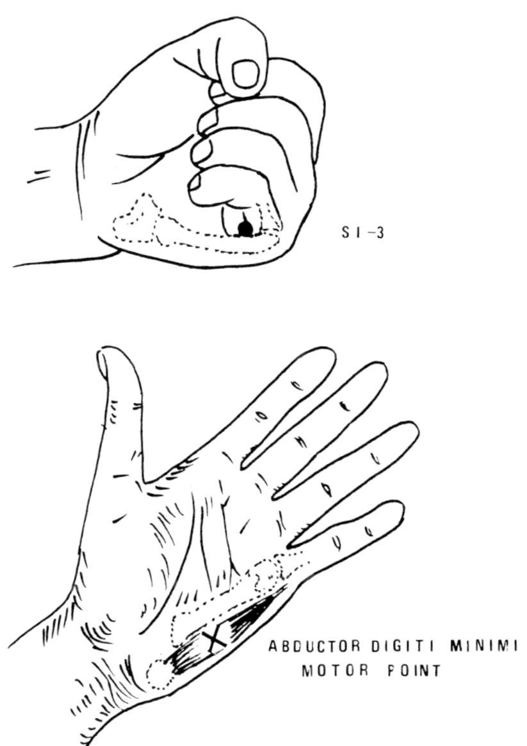

Figure 22 M.

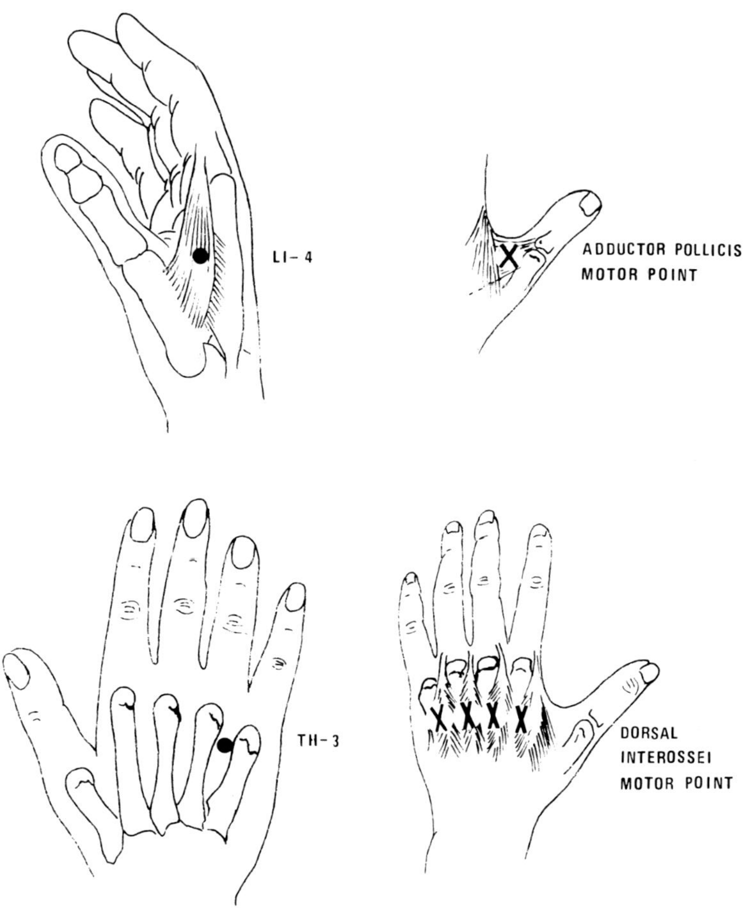
LI-4
ADDUCTOR POLLICIS
MOTOR POINT
TH-3
DORSAL
INTEROSSEI
MOTOR POINT

Figure 22 N.

TABLE II (Cont'd.)

BACK

REGION	NAME	ANATOMICAL LOCATION	PHYSIOLOGIC JUSTIFICATION
Para T_2-T_3	BL-12	Erector spinae muscles 3 cm from midline para T_2-T_3	Erector spinae motor point
Para T_3-T_4	BL-13	Erector spinae muscles 3 cm from midline para T_3-T_4	Erector spinae motor point
Para T_5	BL-15	One fingerbreath lateral to the inferior end of the spinous process of the 5th thoracic vertebra	Erector spinae motor point
Para T_7-T_8	BL-17	Erector spinae muscles 3 cm from midline para T_7-T_8	Lower trapezius motor point
Para T_9-T_{10}	BL-18	Erector spinae muscles 3 cm from midline para T_9-T_{10}	Lower trapezius motor point
Para T_{10}-T_{11}	BL-19	Erector spinae muscles 3 cm from midline para T_{10}-T_{11}	Lower trapezius motor point
Para T_{11}-T_{12}	BL-20	Erector spinae muscles 3 cm from midline para T_{11}-T_{12}	Lower trapezius motor point
Para T_{12}-L_1	BL-21	Erector spinae muscles 3 cm from midline para T_{12}-L_1	Lower trapezius motor point
Para L_2-L_3	BL-23	Erector spinae muscles 3 cm from midline para L_2-L_3	Lower trapezius motor point
Para L_4-L_5	BL-25	Erector spinae muscles 3 cm from midline para L_4-L_5	Erector spinae motor point
Para L_5-S_1	BL-26	Erector spinae muscles 3 cm from midline para L_5-S_1	Erector spinae motor point

(Back Cont'd.)

TABLE II (Cont'd.)

REGION	NAME	ANATOMICAL LOCATION	PHYSIOLOGIC JUSTIFICATION
Para S_1-S_2	BL-27	Erector spinae muscles 3 cm from midline para S_1-S_2	Erector spinae motor point
Para S_2-S_3	BL-28	Erector spinae muscles 3 cm from midline para S_2-S_3	Erector spinae motor point
Mid-Back	BL-40	Between sixth and seventh thoracic vertebrae three inches from mid-line	Trapezius motor point
Sacral Region	BL-49	Level of fourth sacral foramen three inches from midline	Gluteus maximus motor point

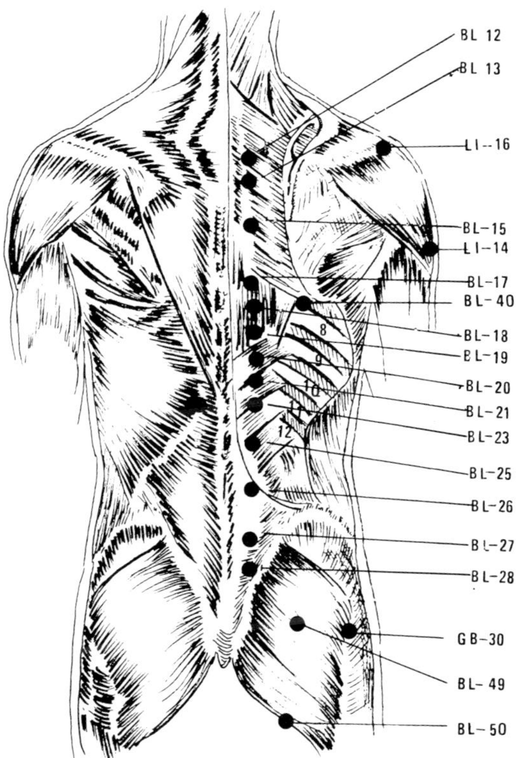
BL 12
BL 13
LI--16
BL-15
LI-14
BL-17
BL-40
8
BL-18
BL-19
9
BL-20
10
BL-21
11
BL-23
12
BL-25
BL-26
BL-27
BL-28
GB-30
BL-49
BL-50

Figure 22 O.

TABLE II (Cont'd.)

LOWER EXTREMITY

REGION	NAME	ANATOMICAL LOCATION	PHYSIOLOGIC JUSTIFICATION
Posterior Trochanter	GB-30	Four fingerbreaths posterior to greater trochanter	Lateral cutaneous nerve of the thigh L2-L3
Midgluteal Crease	BL-50	Midline on gluteal fold	Posterior cutaneous nerve of the thigh S3-S4
Posterior Mid-Thigh	BL-51	Posterior mid-thigh	Posterior cutaneous nerve of the thigh S3-S4
Lateral Mid-Thigh	GB-31	Standing erect, where tip of long finger reaches lateral thigh	Lateral femoral cutaneous n.
Anterior Mid-Thigh	ST-32	5 fingerbreaths superior to the upper margin of patella along the line joining the lateral margin of the patella with the anterior superior iliac spine	Femoral n. posterior division lumbar plexus, L_2, L_3, L_4
Medial Supra Patella	SP-10	Three fingerbreaths above upper pole of patella over vastus medialis	Vastus femoral cutaneous n.
Median Popliteal Crease	BL-54	Middle of popliteal fossa	Posterior femoral cutaneous n. S_2
Lateral Upper Tibialis	ST-36	Four fingerbreaths below lower pole at patella and two fingerbreaths lateral	Tibialis anterior motor point
Anterior Upper Fibula	GB-34	Neck of fibula	Peroneus longus motor point

(Lower Extremity Cont'd.)

TABLE II (Cont'd)

REGION	NAME	ANATOMICAL LOCATION	PHYSIOLOGIC JUSTIFICATION
Mid-Gastrocnemius	BL-57	Junction of medial and lateral heads of gastrocnemius in mid-calf at origin of Achilles tendon	Sural n.
Lower Tibia	SP-6	Four fingerbreaths above medial malleolus	Soleus motor point
Posterior Lateral Malleolus	BL-60	Between Achilles' tendon and lateral malleolus	Flexor hallicus longus motor point
Posterior Median Malleolus	KI-3	Between Achilles' tendon and medial malleolus	Superficial branch of saphenous n. L_3-L_4
Second-Third Metatarsal	ST-44	One fingerbreath proximal to web margin between second and third metatarsals	Superficial peroneal n. (L_5, S_1); lateral plantar n. ($L_{4,5}$, $S1, 2,3$)
First Metatarsal	LV-3	2 cm proximal to web margin between first and second metatarsals on dorsum	Deep peroneal n. (L4,5 S1) medial plantar n. ($L_{4,5}S_{1,2,3}$)
Sole of Foot	KI-1	Between second and third metatarsals on sole of foot	Medial plantar n.
Below Medial Malleolus	KI-6	Internal side of leg 2 cm below the internal malleolus	Medial branches from the tibial nerve

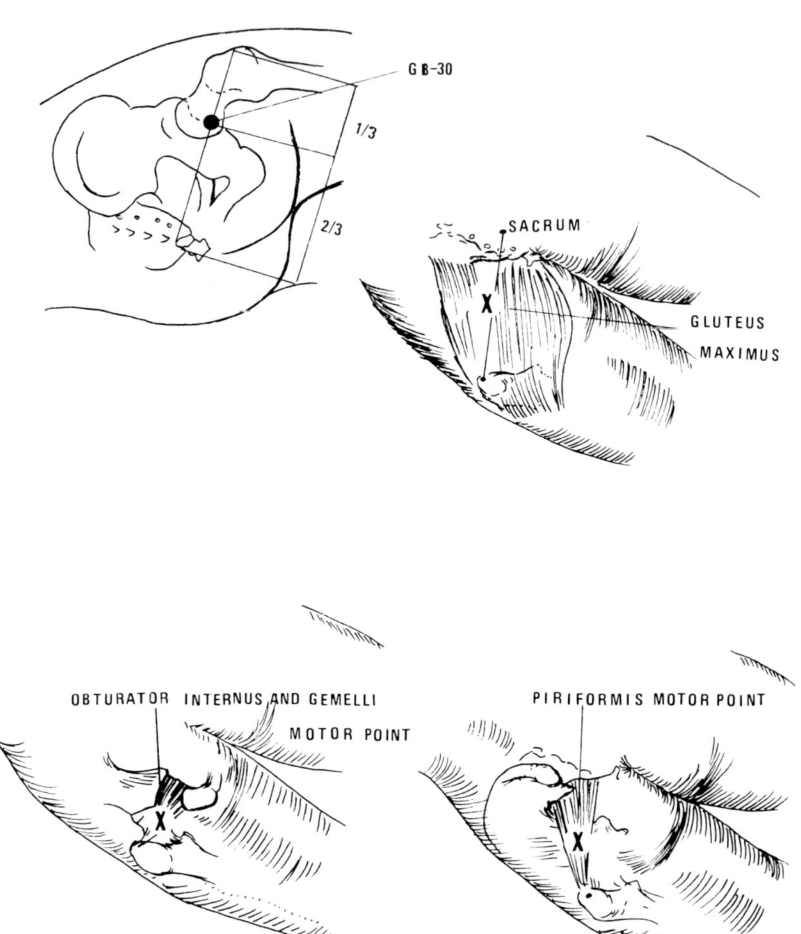
GB-30
1/3
2/3
SACRUM
GLUTEUS
MAXIMUS
OBTURATOR INTERNUS AND GEMELLI
MOTOR POINT
PIRIFORMIS MOTOR POINT

Figure 22 P.

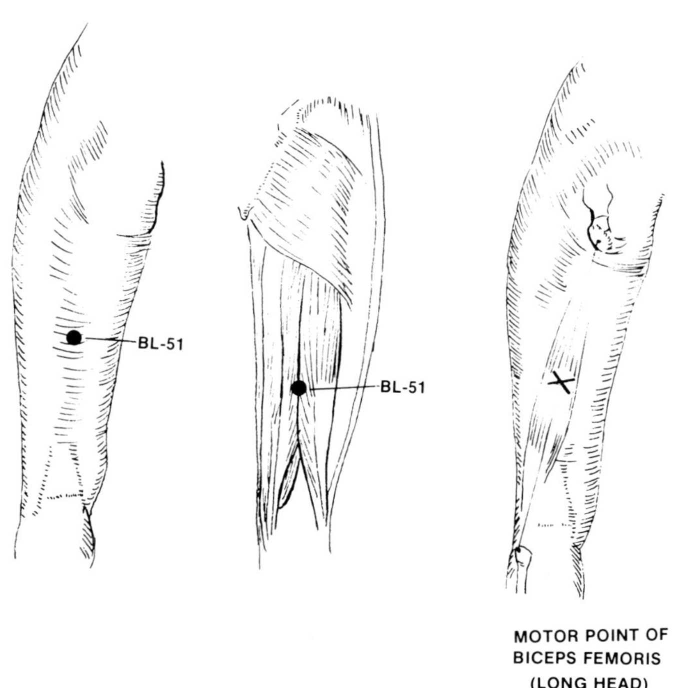

Figure 22 Q.

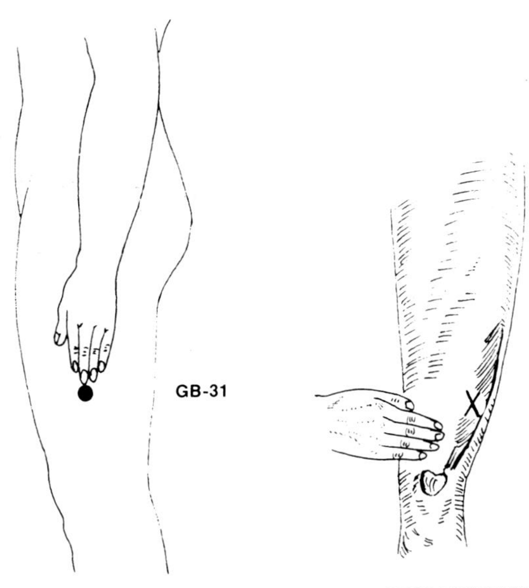

Figure 22 R.

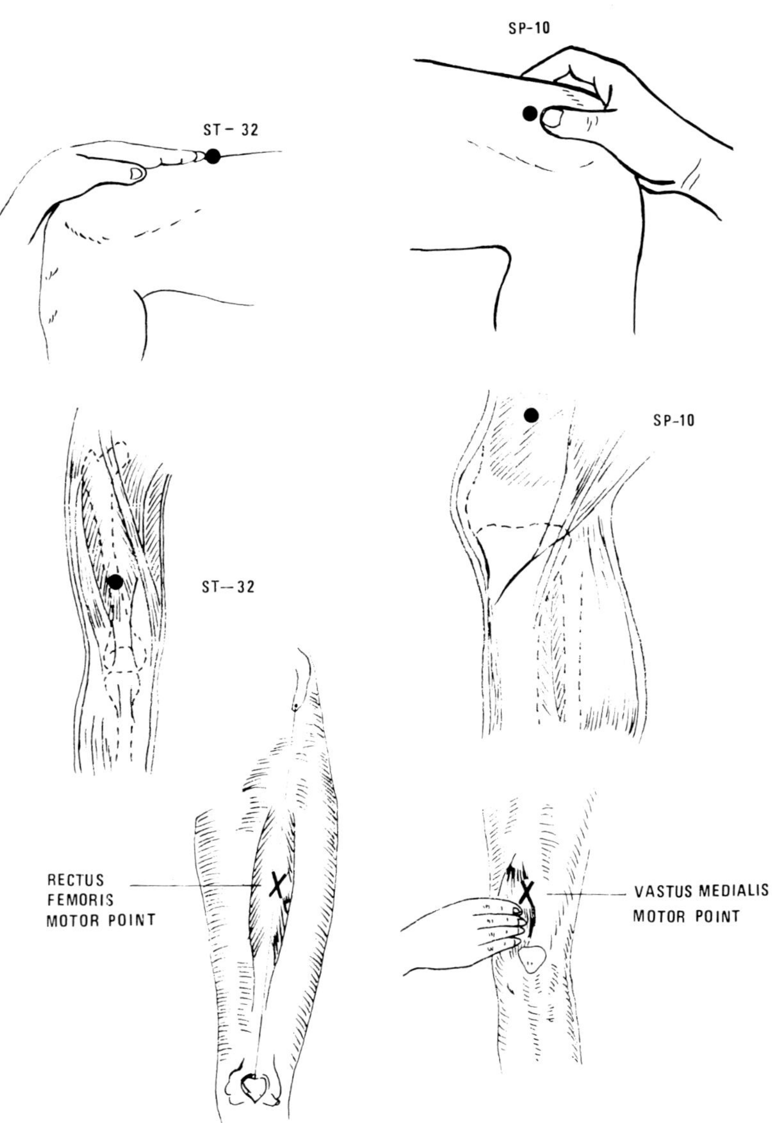
SP-10
ST - 32
SP-10
ST—32
RECTUS
FEMORIS
MOTOR POINT
VASTUS MEDIALIS
MOTOR POINT

Figure 22 S.

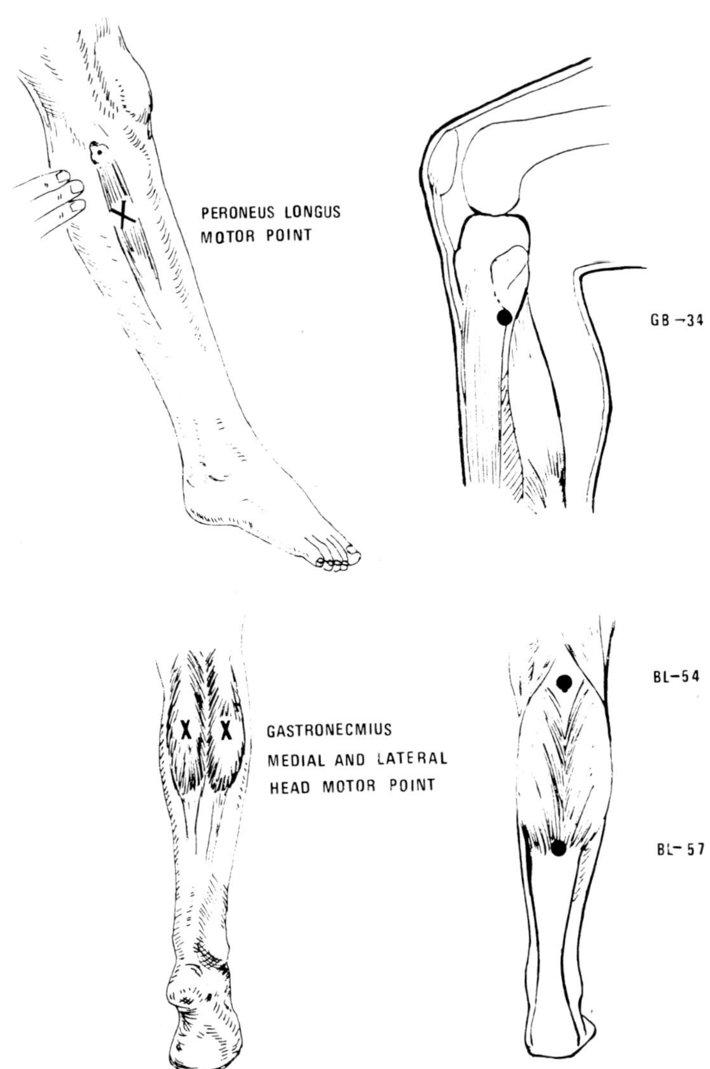
PERONEUS LONGUS
MOTOR POINT
GB -34
GASTRONECMIUS
MEDIAL AND LATERAL
HEAD MOTOR POINT
BL-54
BL-57

Figure 22 T.

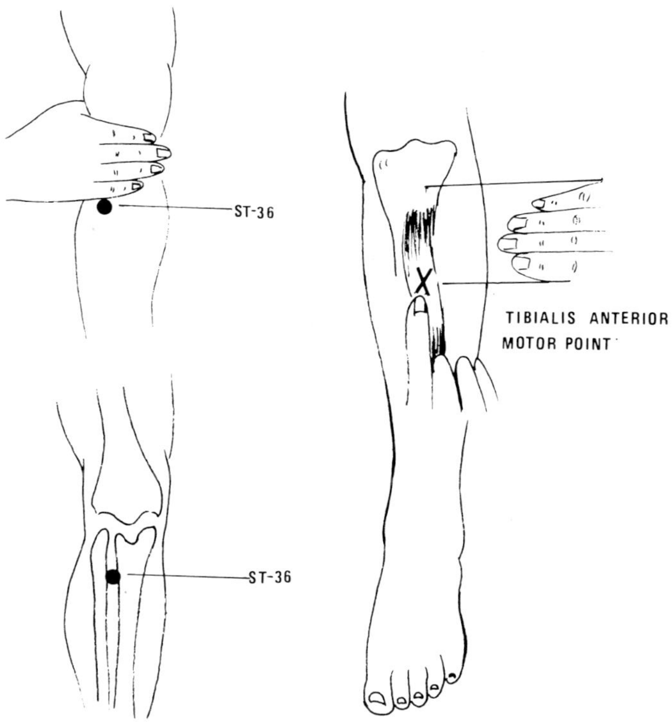

Figure 22 U.

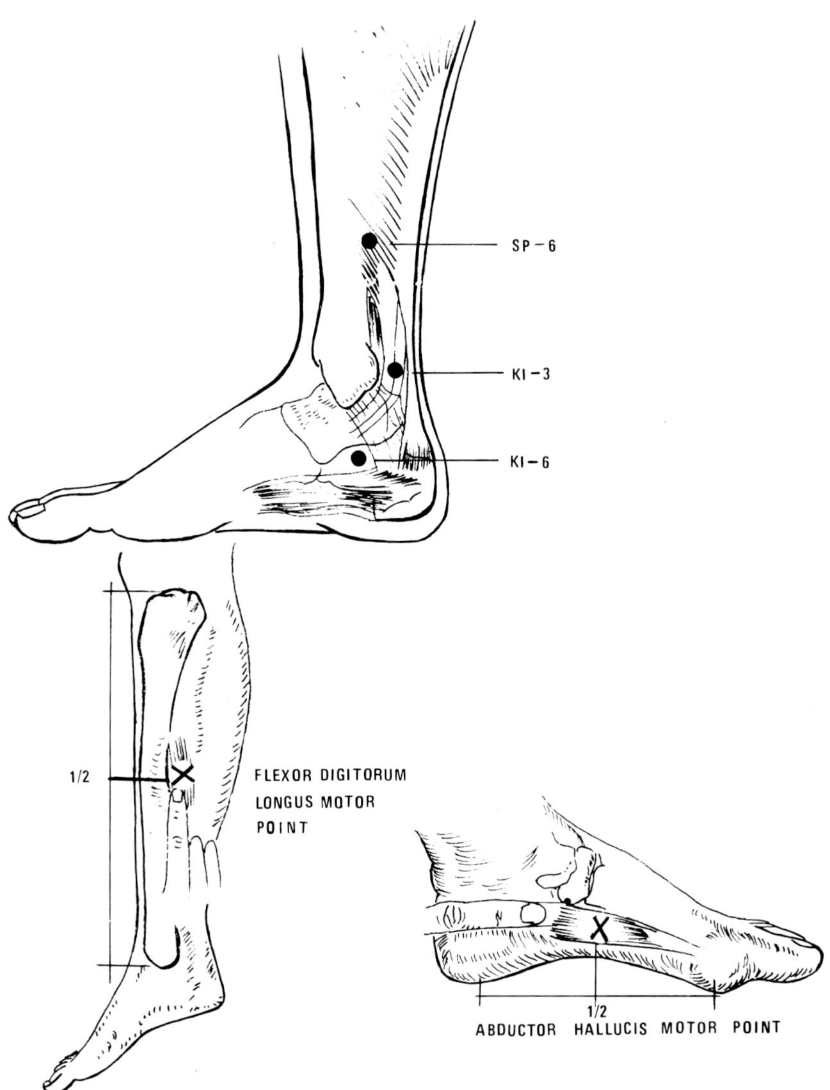
SP – 6
KI – 3
KI – 6
1/2
FLEXOR DIGITORUM
LONGUS MOTOR
POINT
1/2
ABDUCTOR HALLUCIS MOTOR POINT

Figure 22 V.

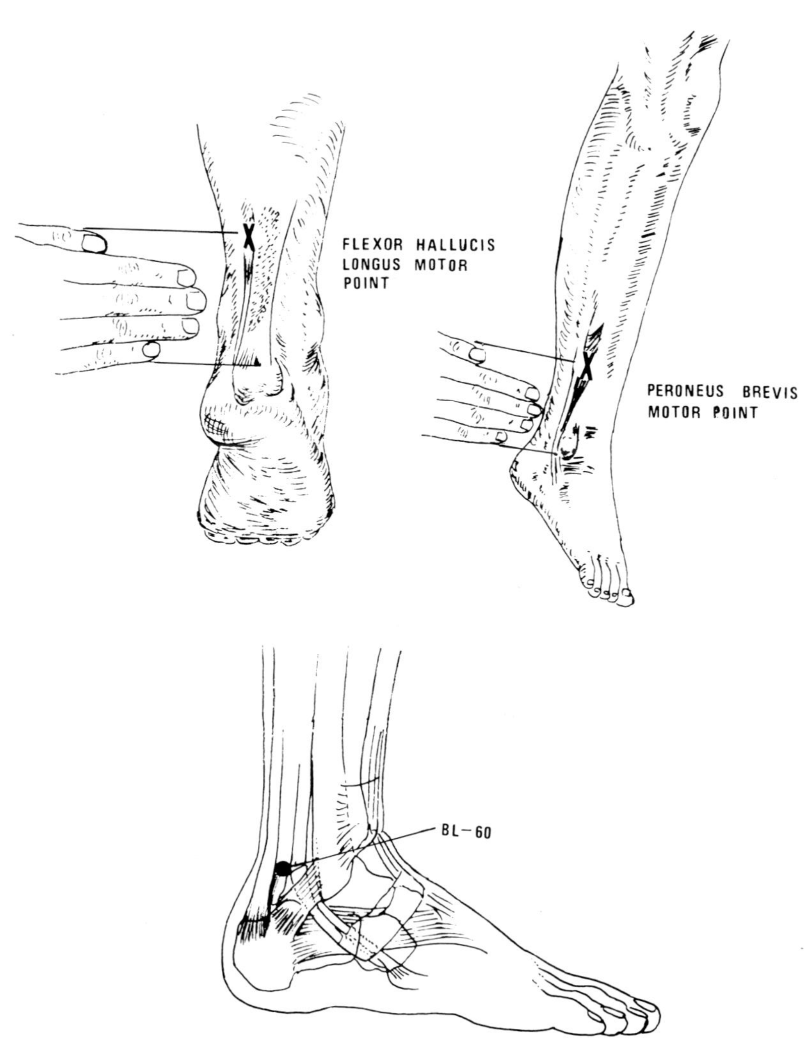
FLEXOR HALLUCIS
LONGUS MOTOR
POINT
PERONEUS BREVIS
MOTOR POINT
BL-60

Figure 22 W.

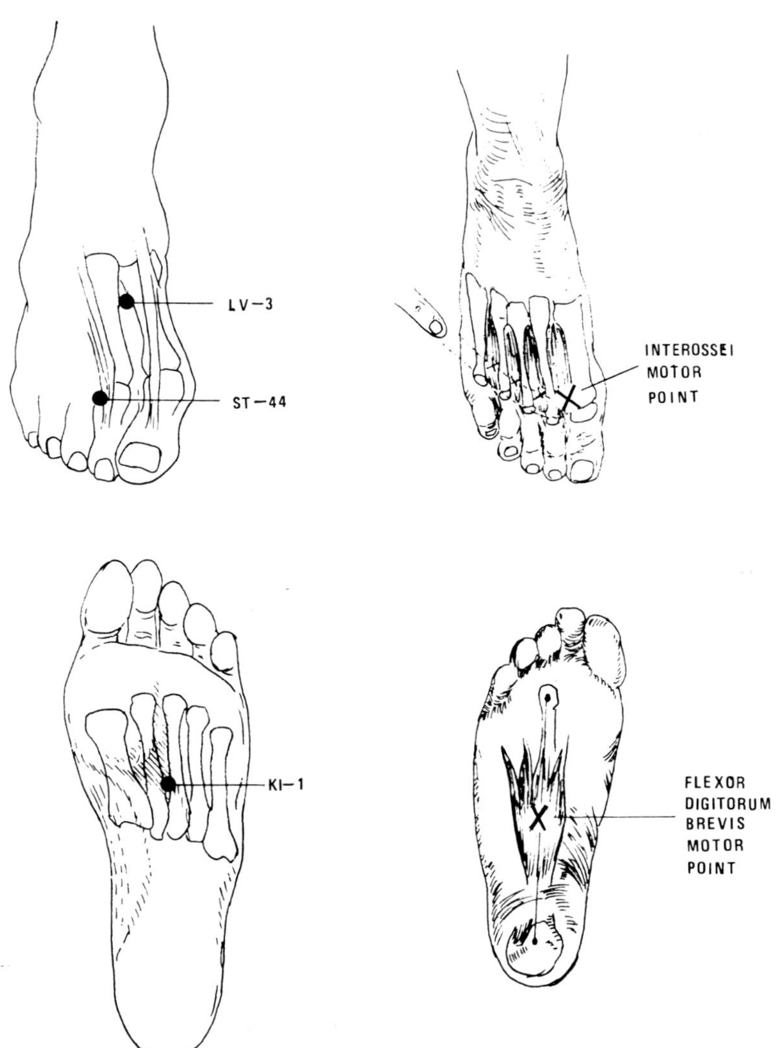
LV-3
ST-44
INTEROSSEI
MOTOR
POINT
KI-1
FLEXOR
DIGITORUM
BREVIS
MOTOR
POINT

Figure 22 X.

Figure 23 (a-g) is a chart of reference for motor point location over the total surface of the body. This gives a general idea of their widespread nature and, illustrates how affliction of any part of the body can be readily treated by points located nearby.

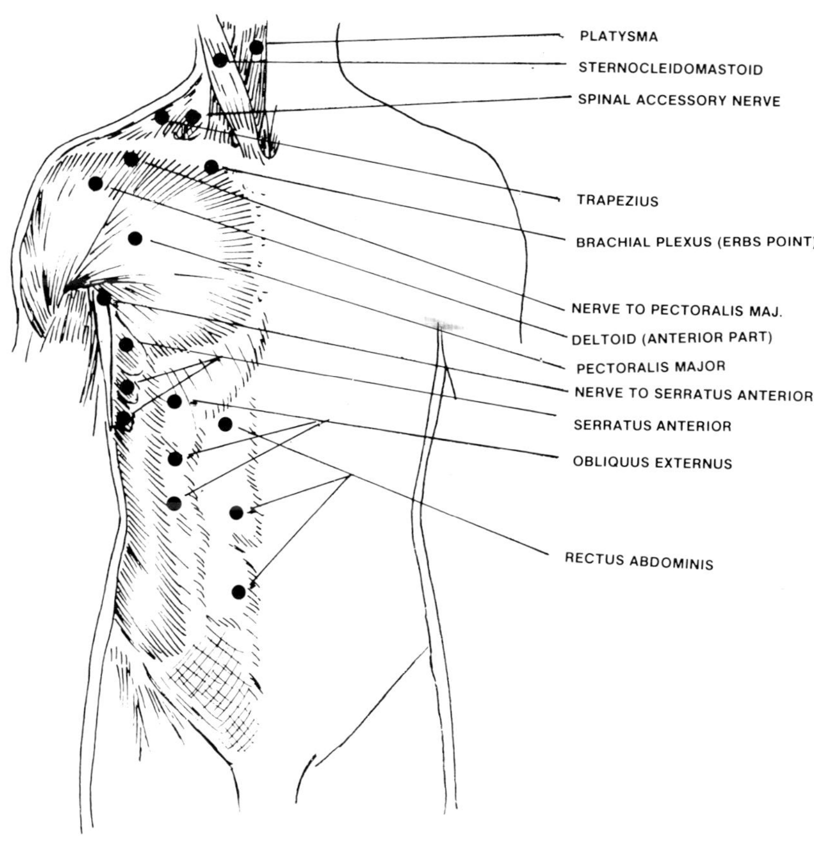

Figure 23. Charts of motor point location.

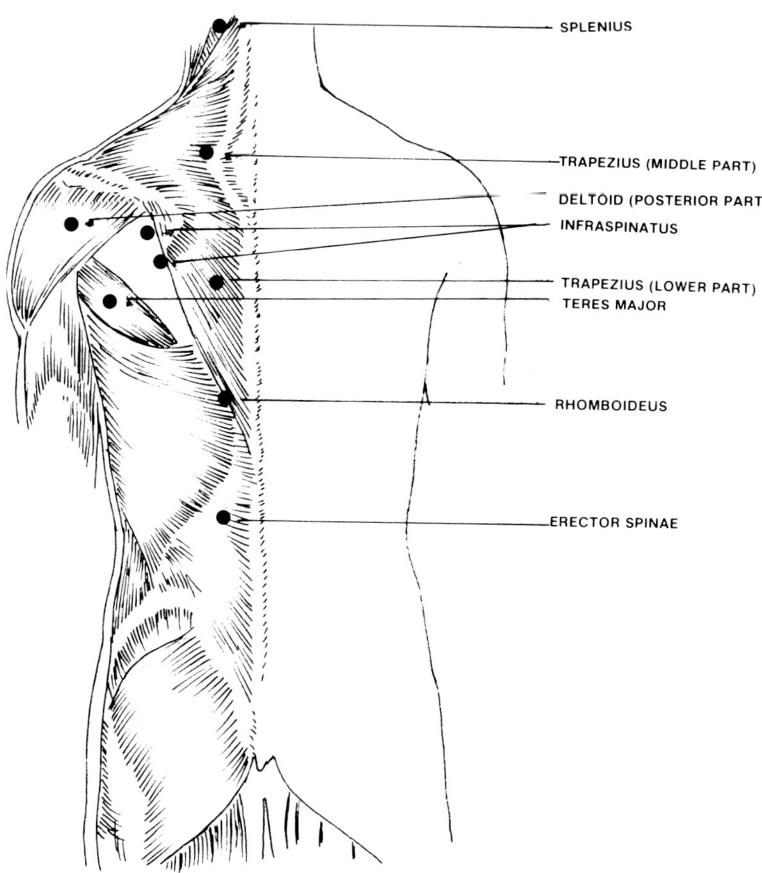

MOTOR POINTS

Figure 23 B.

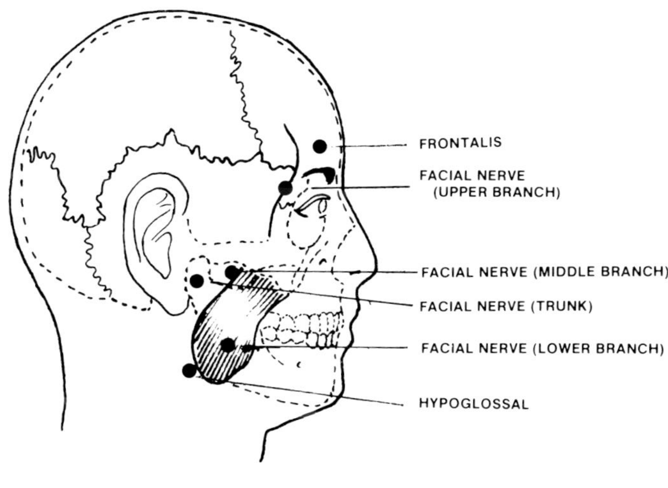

MOTOR POINTS
Figure 23 C.

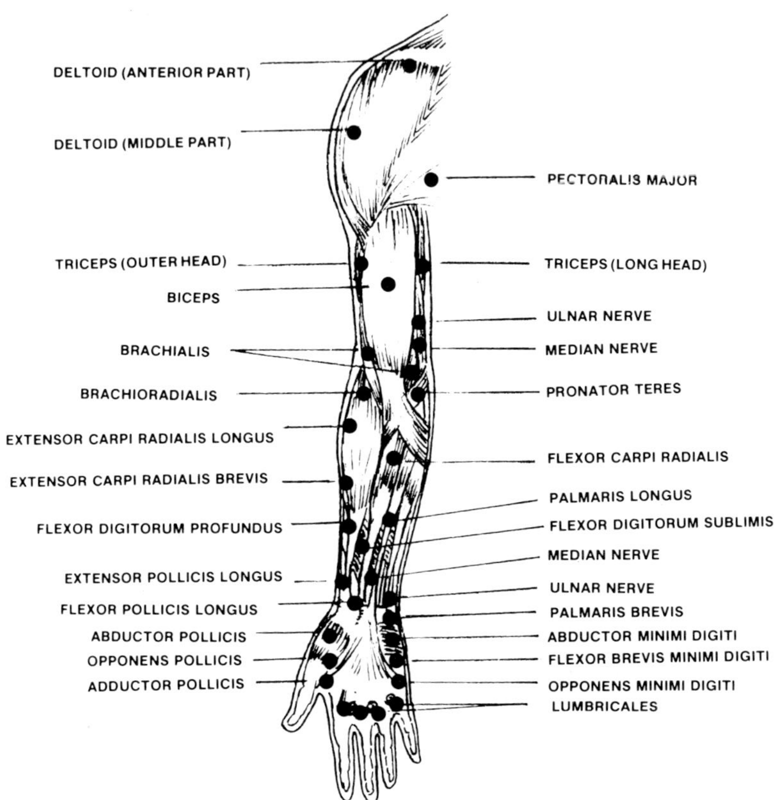

MOTOR POINTS

Figure 23 D.

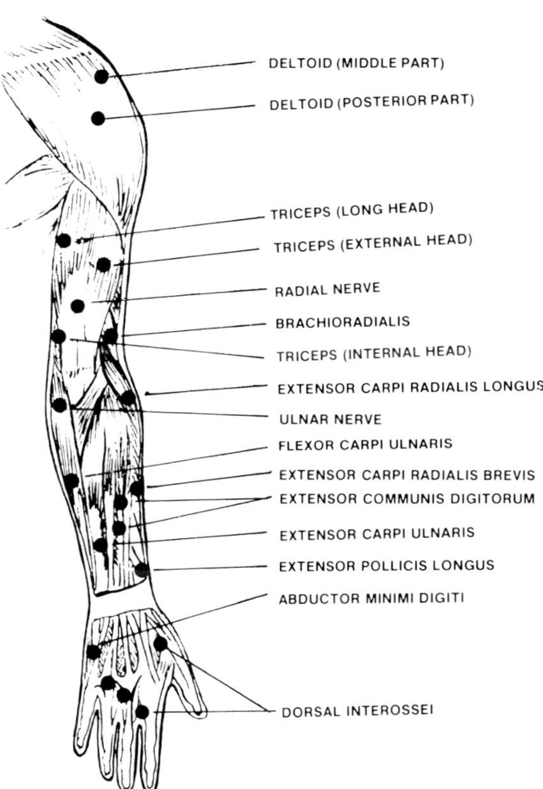

MOTOR POINTS

Figure 23 E.

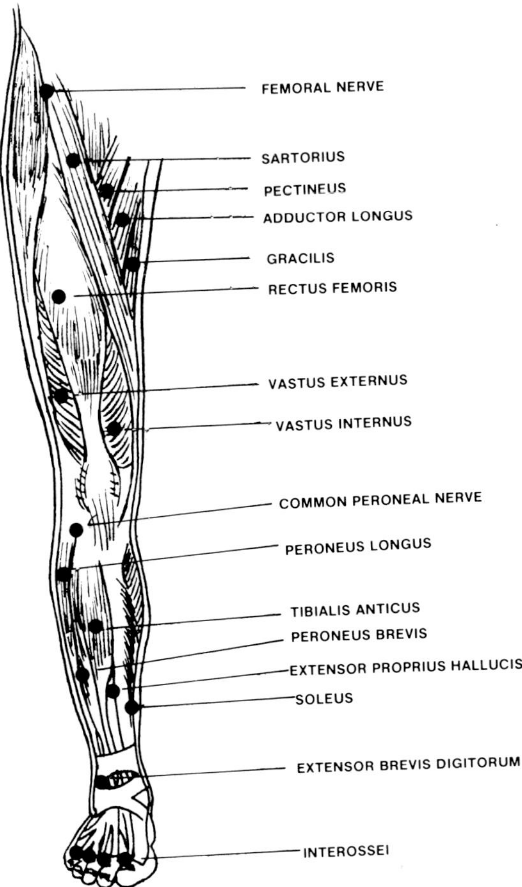

MOTOR POINTS

Figure 23 F.

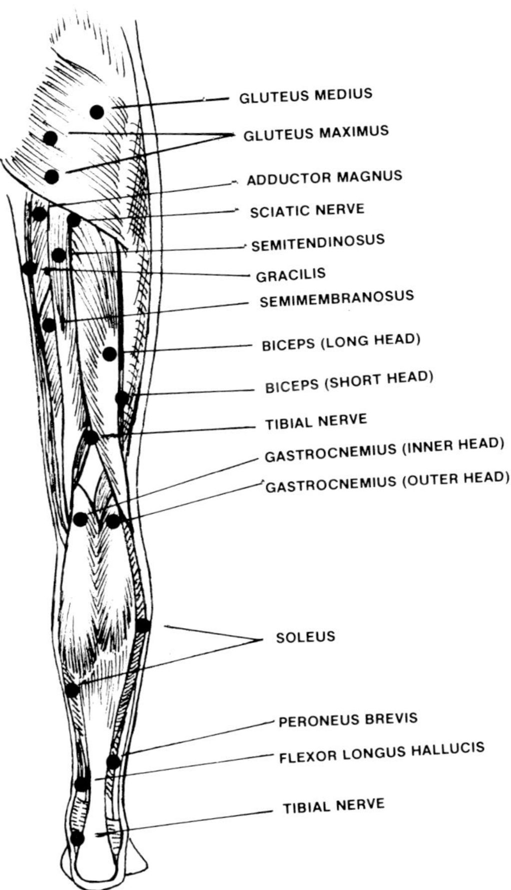

MOTOR POINTS

Figure 23 G.

We have preserved the original two letter abbreviation of the meridian designation for those points that are either identical with or lie near motor points. It seemed wise to stay with this traditional designation of acupuncture points as we did not see any gain in confusing an already confused literature with yet another system of point nomenclature. Table III lists the abbreviations we have selected to describe the points we use.

TABLE III

POINT-MERIDIAN DESIGNATIONS USED IN THIS BOOK

	Abbreviation	Meridian
Bilateral	LU	Lung
	LI	Large intestine
	ST	Stomach
	SP	Spleen
	HE	Heart
	SI	Small intestine
	BL	Bladder
	KI	Kidney
	PC	Pericardium
	TH	Triple heater
	GB	Gall bladder
	LV	Liver
Unpaired	GV	Governing vessel
	CV	Conception vessel
	EM	"extra meridian" Points not located on meridians

B. SELECTION OF POINTS ACCORDING TO NEUROTOME DISTRIBUTION

Previous sections have discussed the Gate theory of Melzak and Wall, as well as observations of Gunn on alterations in nerve function attendant upon root or nerve compression, utilizing concepts from Cannon's Law of Denervation. The pain mechanisms to be controlled by treatment visualized from such points of view would seem amenable to therapeutic manipulation either within the troubled neurotome or its corresponding myotome, dermatome, sclerotome or sympathetic ramus. It is only necessary, first, to appraise the extent of the pain and locate the appropriate spinal segment involved.

Effective points for the treatment of many conditions, therefore, will be found on the dorsal surface of the body, on either side of the vertebral column, approximately 1½ inches lateral to the midline and at the level of each intervertebral foramen at the point where the spinal nerve exits between the vertebrae. These correspond approximately to those meridian points called "bladder points" (BL) in traditional Chinese acupuncture (Figure 24). It is probable that the greatest effect of stimulation here is through muscle afferents of the posterior rami of the spinal nerves. According to the position and depth of placement, needles here will pierce the long muscles of the back (longissimus dorsi and spinalis dorsi) and may reach motor points of the semi-spinalis and multifidus muscles (Figure 25). Depending upon the strength of electrical stimulus the main entering nerve trunks (posterior and anterior rami), may be stimulated directly. The thickness of the muscle mass here makes it exceedingly unlikely (save with extremely deep penetration) that the peritoneal or thoracic cavities would be inadvertently penetrated.

Figure 26 illustrates that the palpated vertebral spine does not, in all cases, quite correspond to the vertebral body or the spinal nerve root of the same number. It will be recalled that as one descends the spinal cord, the nerve roots angle sharply and must travel longer distances from the shortened cord to the point of their exit from the intervertebral foramina.

Upon entering the spinal cord, afferent impulses from peripheral nerves may synapse directly for reflex arc function or may ascend or descend a few segments. It can, thus, often be useful to place needles above or below the neural level of the lesion either to augment the primary stimulus or when it is necessary to avoid a skin area that may be infected, scarred or otherwise inaccessible to use.

Stimulation of the points on the side opposite to the lesion can be effective due to the fact that some fibers cross the spinal cord at or close to the level of the lesion. The ancient acupuncturist took notice of such effects. Thus, there is a saying in the Chinese literature on acupuncture that states: "shoot a bow to the right and to the left to send two arrows at the same time." Such stimulation can be blocked by lesions of the cord for in hemiplegic patients stimulation of LI-4 and ST-36 on the side of the lesion failed to produce the rise in pain threshold seen following stimulation of corresponding points on the normal side (102). A similar mechanism in patients with paraplegia blocked the analgesic effect of stimulation at ST-36 on the legs while this lesion did not interfere with the effect of stimulating LI-4 on the hands.

The importance of segmental neurotome relations has been well illustrated by Chang of Shanghai (103). He demonstrated that stimulation of an acupuncture point which lies at the midpoint of the sterno-cleido-mastoid muscle (also its motor point) produces analgesia sufficient for

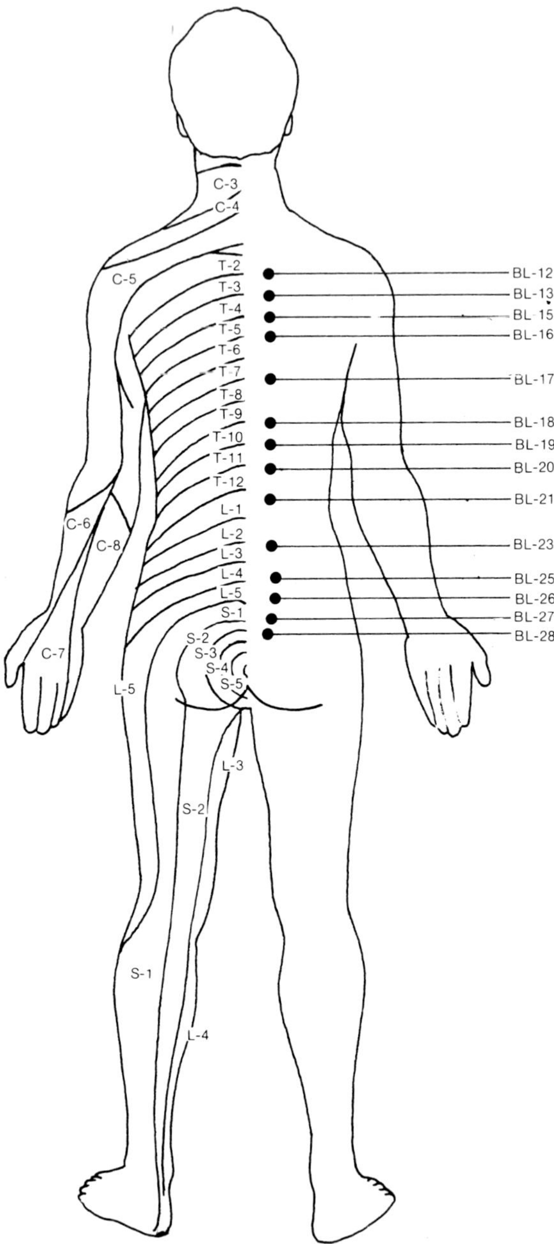

Figure 24. Correspondence of acupuncture meridian "bladder" points to spinal neurotome distribution.

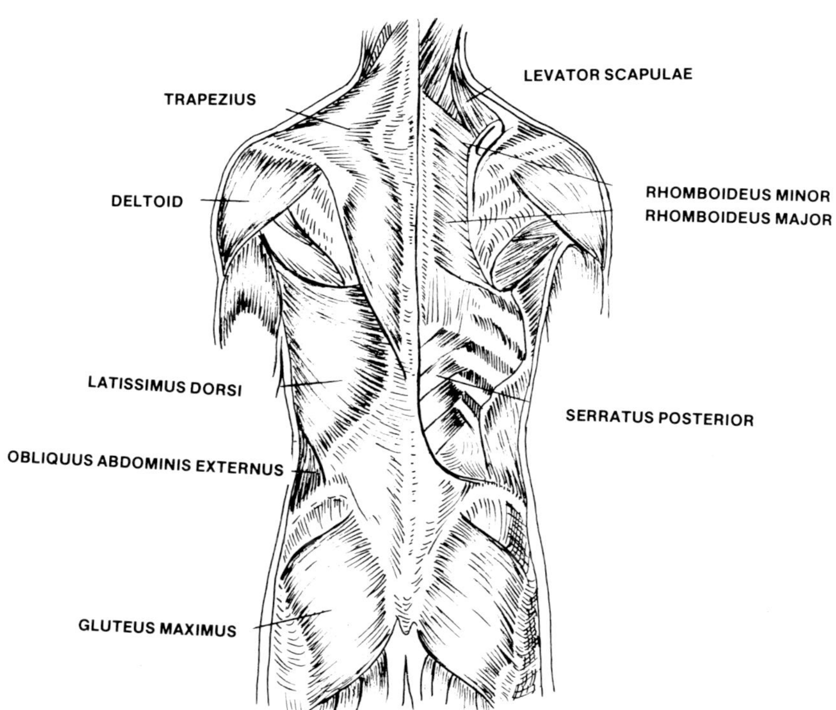

Figure 25. (a) Anatomy of paravertebral musculature. (b) Cross sections at representative levels of the body indicating approximate thickness of muscle mass as a guide for depth of needle insertion.

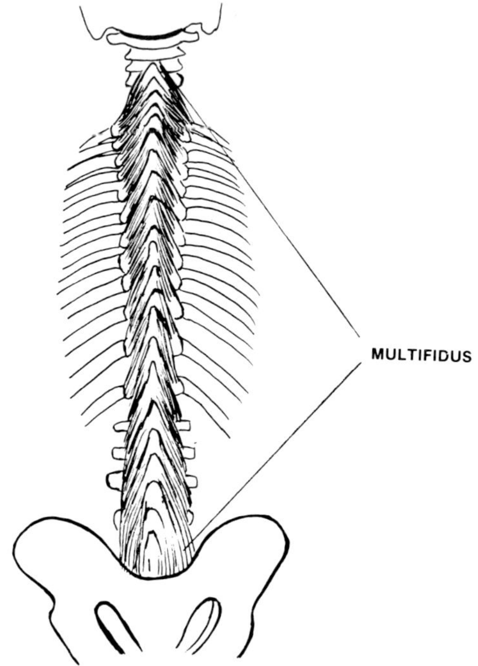

DEEP MUSCLES OF THE BACK

Figure 25 A-2.

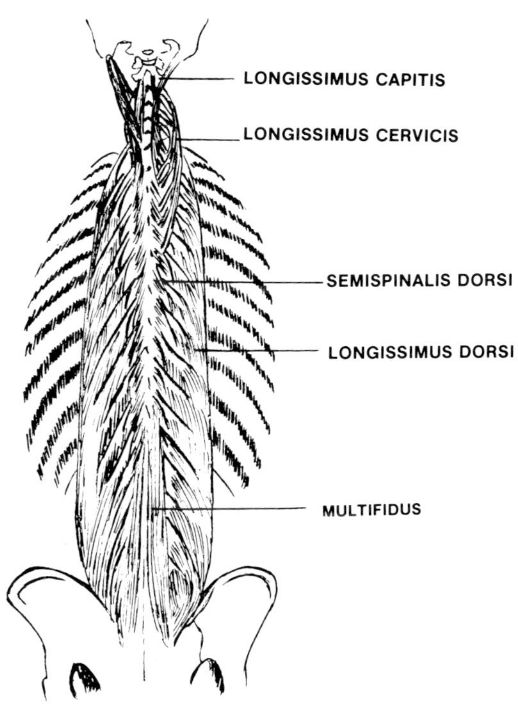

DEEP MUSCLES OF THE BACK

Figure 25 A-3.

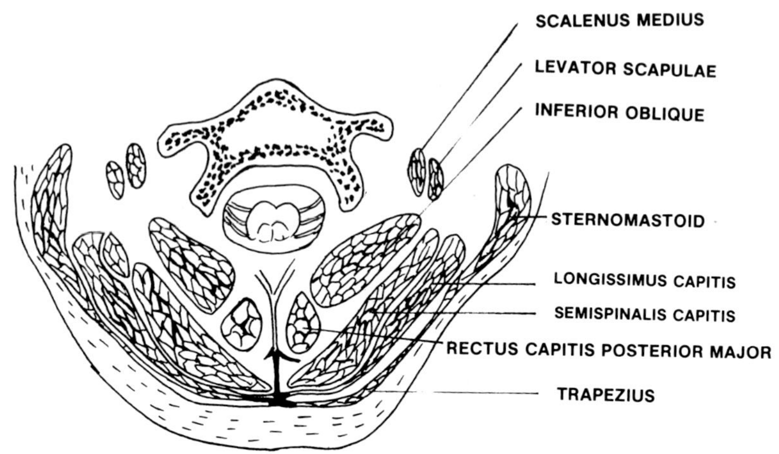

CROSS-SECTION OF THE NUCHAL REGION AT THE LEVELOF THE AXIS

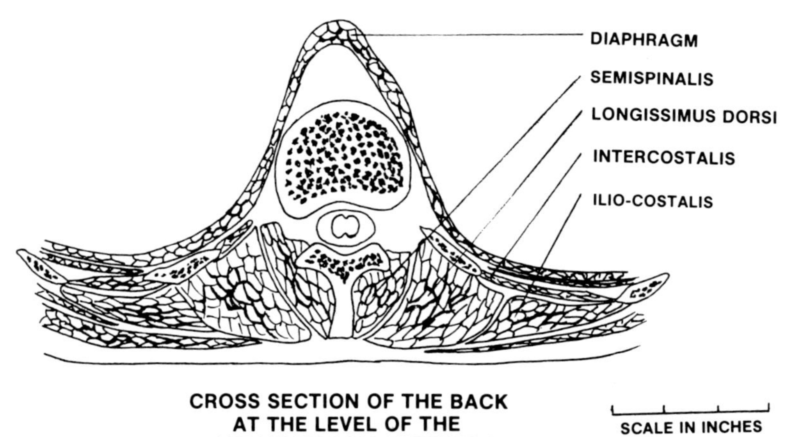

CROSS SECTION OF THE BACK AT THE LEVEL OF THE 12TH THORACIC VERTEBRA

Figure 25 B-1.

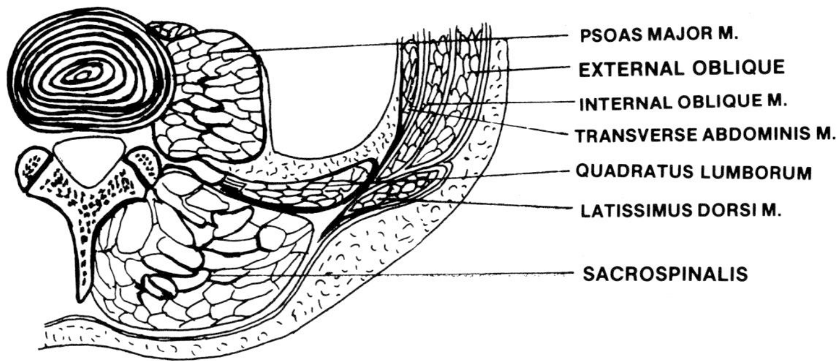

CROSS SECTION OF THE BACK AT THE LEVEL OF THE 2ND LUMBAR VERTEBRA

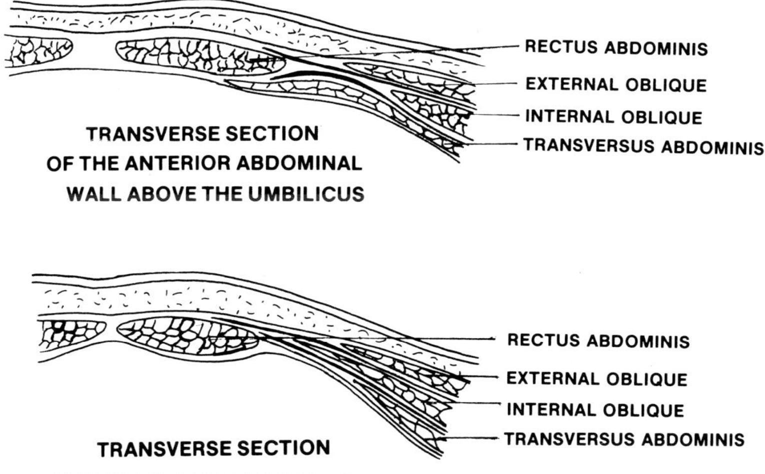

Figure 25 B-2.

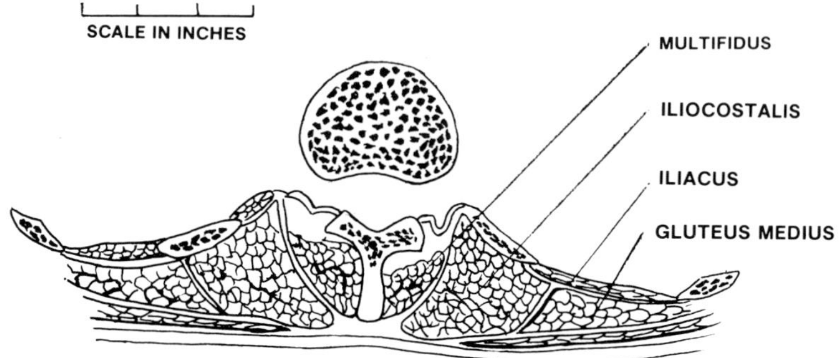

TRANSVERSE SECTION OF THE BACK AT THE LEVEL OF THE 5th LUMBAR VERTEBRA

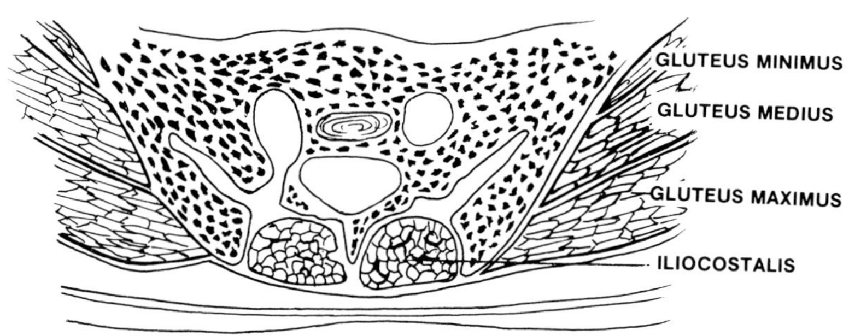

TRANSVERSE SECTION OF THE BACK AT THE LEVEL OF THE SACRAL PROMONTORY

Figure 25 B-3.

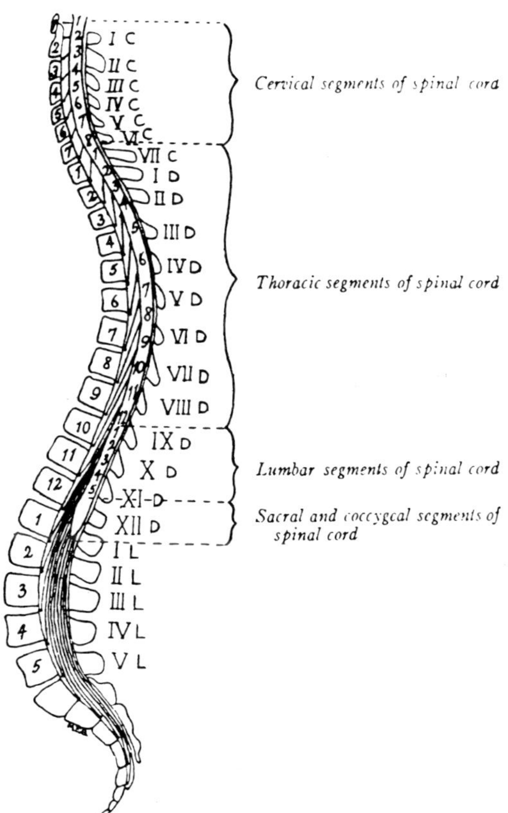

Figure 26. Level of various segments of the spinal cord with reference to the vertebrae. From Ranson, S.W.: *The Anatomy of the Nervous System*. Sixth Edition, Revised 1939. Saunders Publishing Company.

thyroidectomy. This occurs because this cervical nerve (C3) is from the same spinal root that serves the capsule of the thyroid gland.

The same principle can apply to treatment of the face with its sensory innervation distributed over the three branches of the trigeminal nerve: opthalamic, maxillary and mandibular (Figure 27) and with the spinal tract of the trigeminal nerve nucleus reaching downwards to meet ascending impulses from the cervical area.

Figure 28 is a diagram illustrating how neurotomes may overlap. Figure 29 shows diagrams of the neurotome distribution on the surface of the body together with comparable illustrations of dermatome distribution. This makes it clear why an area painful to deep pressure may relate to the spinal segment innervating the underlying muscle (myotome), rather than the spinal segment overlying the afflicted spot (dermatome). Table IV lists the muscles of the upper and lower extremities according to segmental innervation. It may be appropriate to place a needle for stimulation in the tender area or motor point of the affected muscle and, as well, in the paravertebral point of the corresponding neurotome. Such needles should be placed deeply within the muscle tissue. It has long been noted in the acupuncture literature that the most effective treatment occurs when the needle is placed to such depth that needle sensation (a dull ache, throbbing or drawing sensation) is experienced.

At times, it may be appropriate to place needles more superficially to stimulate tender points within the skin or subcutaneous tissue (dermatomes). Electrical stimulation of such dermatome points can produce a counter-irritant effect as seen with stimulation using the flat, superficially applied skin electrodes of TENS (transcutaneous nerve stimulation). In our experience, deeper motor point stimulation has been more useful for the production of lasting effects than is superficial stimulation.

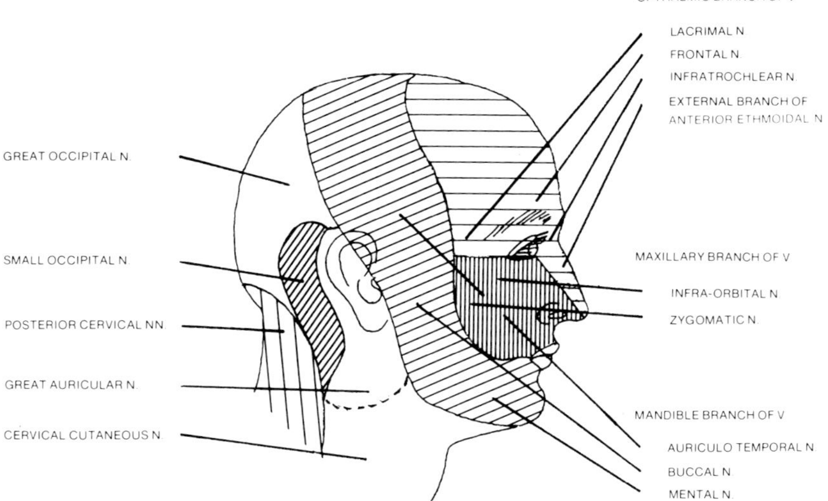

Figure 27. Sensory zones of the head and neck.

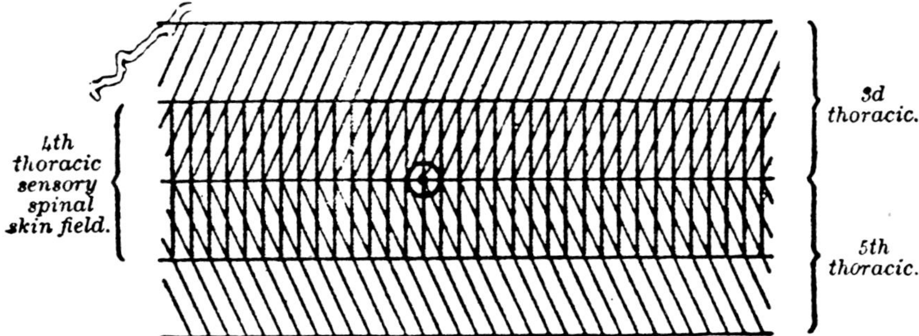

Figure 28. Schematic illustrating the overlap of dermatomes. From Ranson, S.W.: *The Anatomy of the Nervous System*. Sixth Edition. Revised, 1939. Saunders Publishing Company.

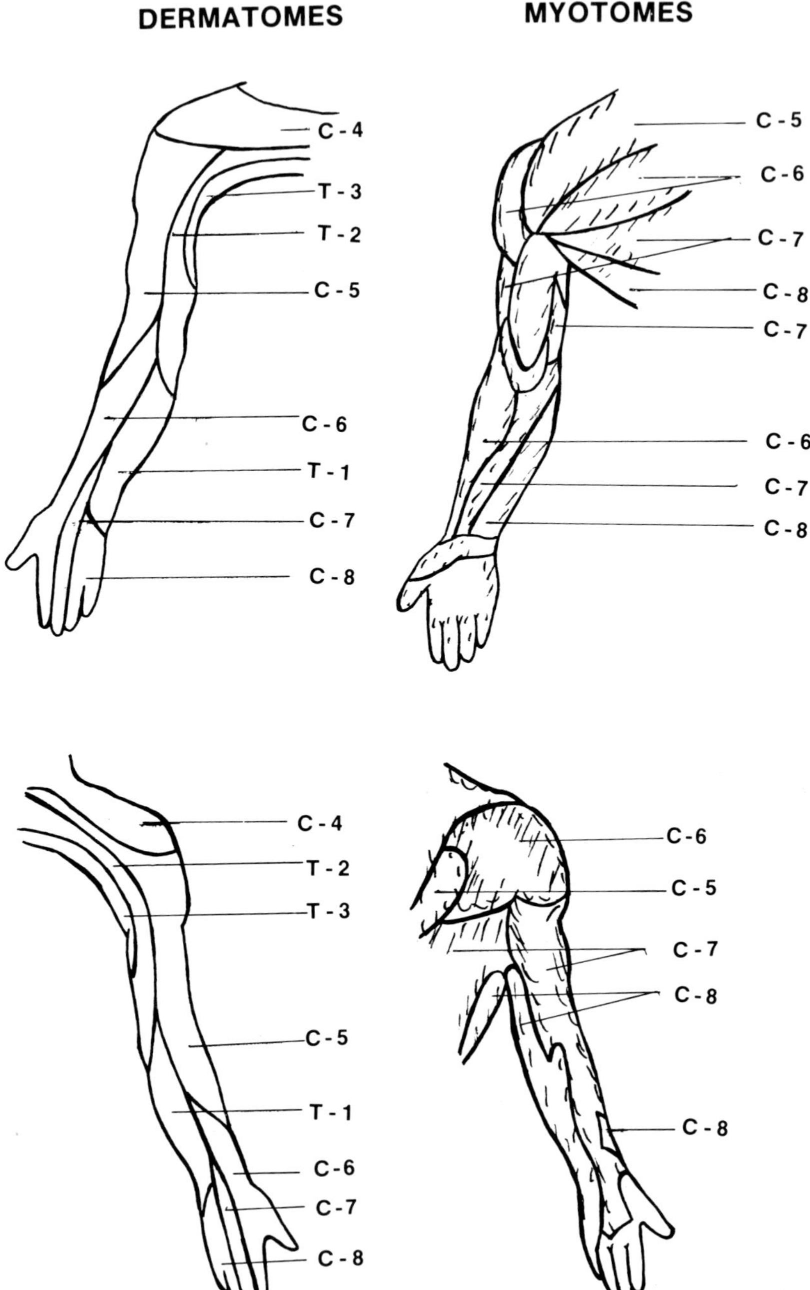

Figure 29. Comparison of myotome and dermatome distribution from corresponding neurotome segments.

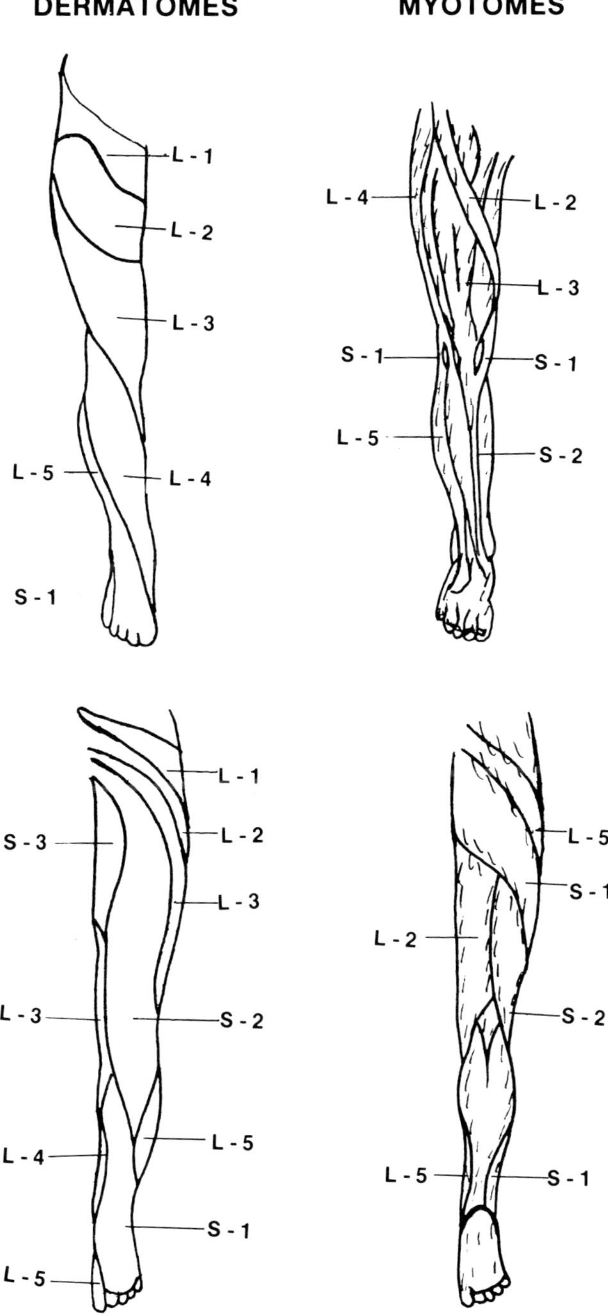
DERMATOMES
MYOTOMES
L - 1
L - 2
L - 3
L - 5
L - 4
S - 1
L - 4
L - 2
L - 3
S - 1
S - 1
L - 5
S - 2
L - 1
S - 3
L - 2
L - 3
L - 3
S - 2
L - 5
L - 4
S - 1
L - 5
L - 5
S - 1
L - 2
S - 2
L - 5
S - 1

Figure 29 B.

TABLE IV(a)

SEGMENTAL INNERVATION OF MUSCLES
OF THE LOWER EXTREMITY

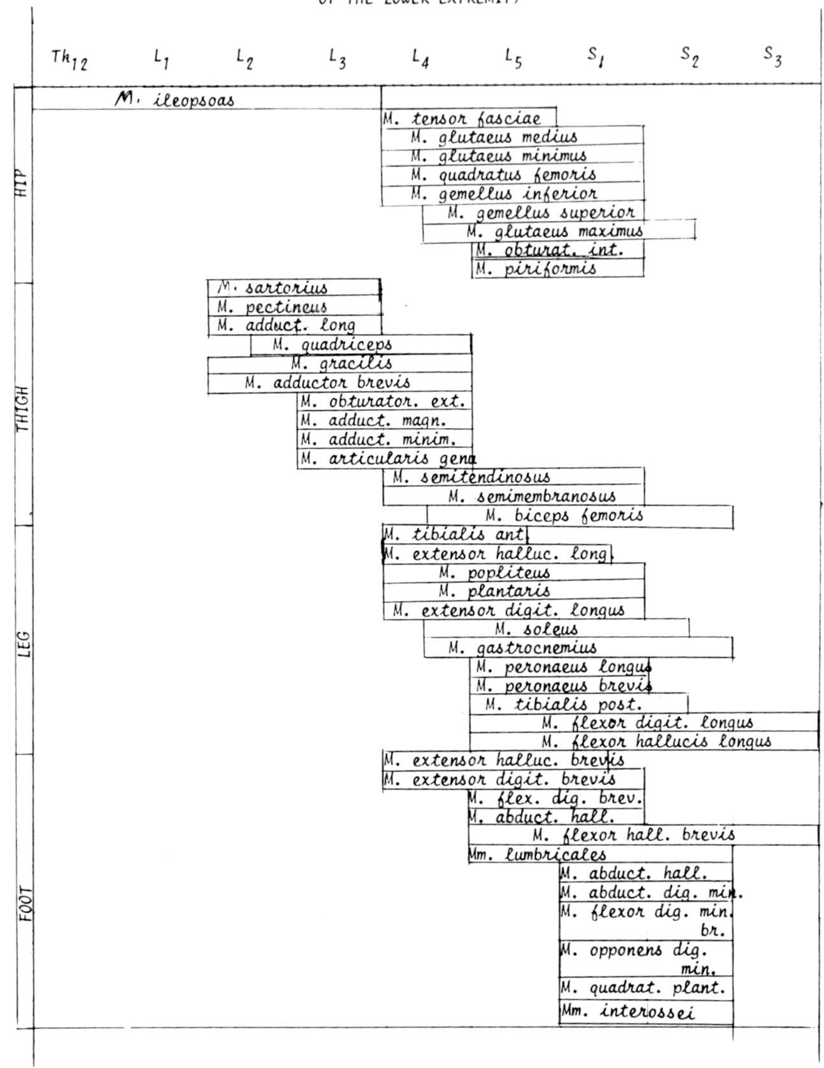

TABLE IV(b)

SEGMENTAL INNERVATION OF MUSCLES
OF THE UPPER EXTREMITY

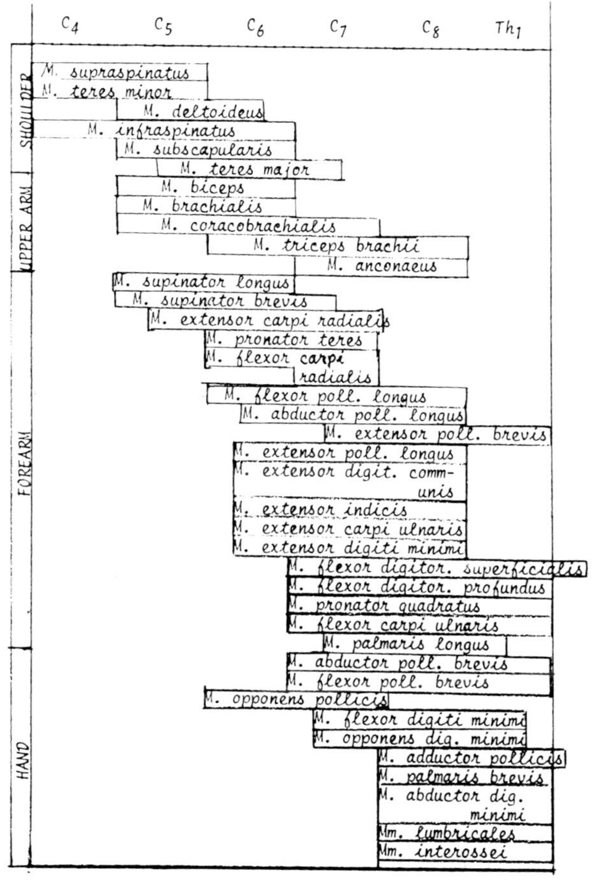

Figure 30 illustrates how pain in certain remote areas can arise from corresponding nerve root irritation. This pattern can, thus, readily serve as the basis for using acupuncture stimulation of a given neurotome as a point of reference for relief of pain in remote, but corresponding dermatome area.

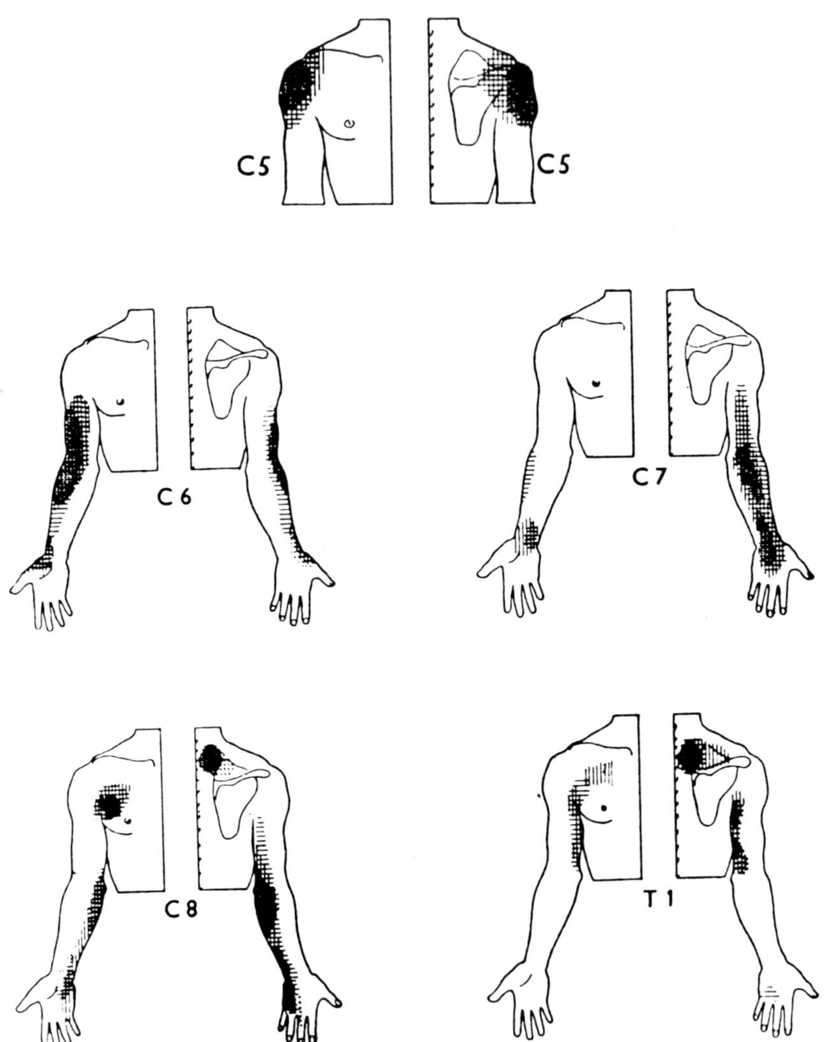

Figure 30. Distribution of pain on the extremities arising from stimulation of interspinous ligaments C_5, C_6, C_7, C_8, T_1 and L_3, L_4, L_5, S_1 and S_2. From Kellgren, J.K.: On the distribution of pain arising from deep somatic structures with charts of segmental pain areas. *Clinical Science*, 1939-42, 4:35-36.

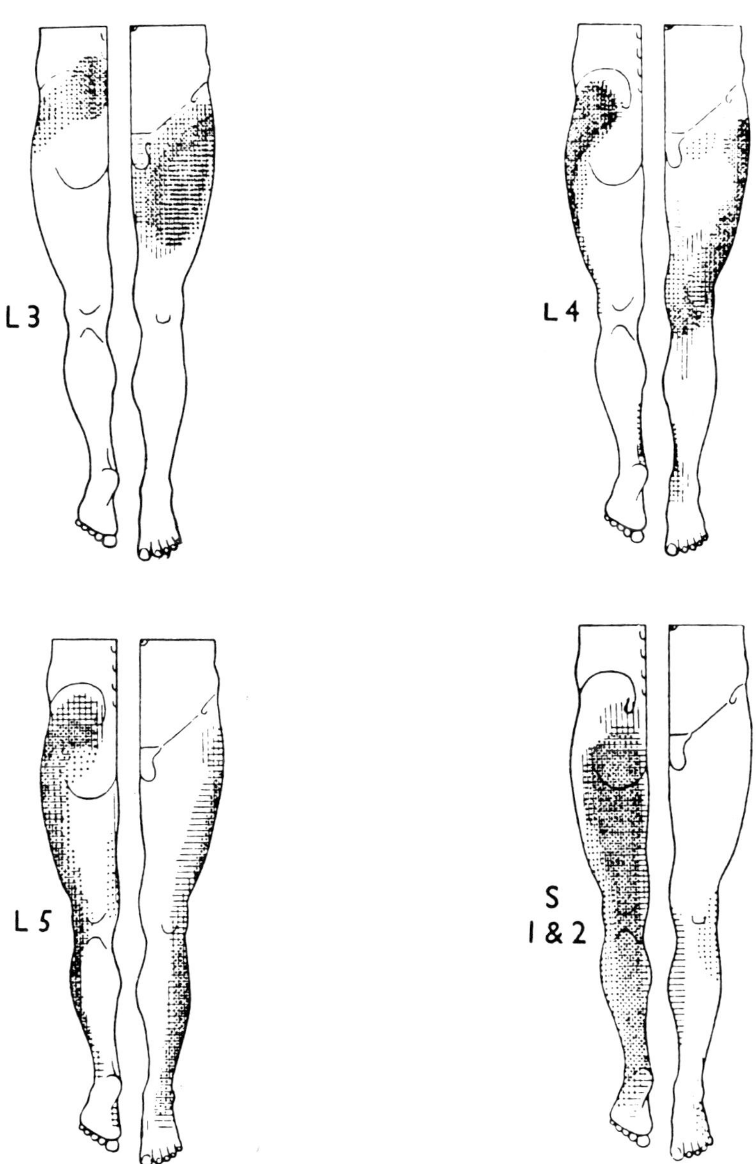

Figure 30 B.

C. CUTANEO-VISCERAL AND VISCERO-CUTANEOUS REFLEX POINTS

Paralleling the paradigm for selection of points for stimulation within neural segments for referred pain from musculo-fascial structures is that for locating points for the treatment of visceral dysfunction. Such points of reference have long been known in medicine. Henry Head in 1893 (87) noted the cutaneously referred pain of visceral disease. He demonstrated that counter irritation over the skin and subcutaneous areas of maximal tenderness could alleviate visceral disturbances. He noted that there was often a bilateral distribution of the pain especially with chronic visceral disturbances. MacKenzie (85) and Kellgran (86), have shown that pain arising from viscera will call into play the cerebrospinal system of sensory nerves with the pain being referred reflexly to the area supplied by the corresponding neurotome. Mann (98), early used the concept of viscero-cutaneous and cutaneo-visceral points to describe the action of some acupuncture points on organs. Weiss and Davis in 1928 (104), noted that referred pain from internally located viscera could be abolished by procaine infiltration of tender areas in the somatic zones of reference, zones that followed patterns often highly consistent from one person to another. Thus, for practical purposes, the segmental distribution of nerves may be of use in selecting effective points for stimulation for the relief of visceral dysfunction.

As disease modifies the function of one organ it may well also affect other organs. This is not only because their functions may interrelate but also because of the spread of neural irritation to adjacent segments up and down the spinal cord. Thus, for example, pain, muscular contractions and vomiting can occur from disturbance of viscera at any of several locations in the body. The segment of spinal cord stimulated by the afferent autonomic fibers from the disturbed viscus can become irritable and produce pain, as well as hyperalgesia of both the skin and the muscles in the external body wall. The area may be remote from the disturbed viscus, lie over it or extend widely around it but in all cases reference to neurotome locations can serve to identify the point for needle placement.

In the living organism there is a succession of stimuli constantly passing from the viscera via afferent nerves to the spinal cord and producing a reflex regulation to maintain homeostasis in muscles, blood vessels, etc. These processes are continually conducted and in such a way that they give rise to no appreciable sensation. If, however, some morbid process occurs in any viscus an imbalance will occur in the homeostatic mechanism. This will change and affect neighboring nerve cells which will induce a reaction of increased muscle tension, and some alteration such as a change in role of function or of internal secretion in associated organ systems. To restore homeostasis it is suggested that the needle for electrostimulation be placed in the dermatome or mytome that corresponds to the nerve supplying the afflicted organ.

Figure 31 shows the correspondence between certain para-vertebrally located acupuncture points and the neurotome segments that innervate body organs. These points (BL points) are ideally situated for stimulation of the dorsal roots carrying afferent impulses from these organs. Figure 32 illustrates the mechanism of referred pain by which such a stimulus from a dysfunctioning organ (splanchnotome) enters the spinal cord and refers as an area of pain on the body wall (dermatome) corresponding to the viscera served by this same spinal cord segment (neurotome).

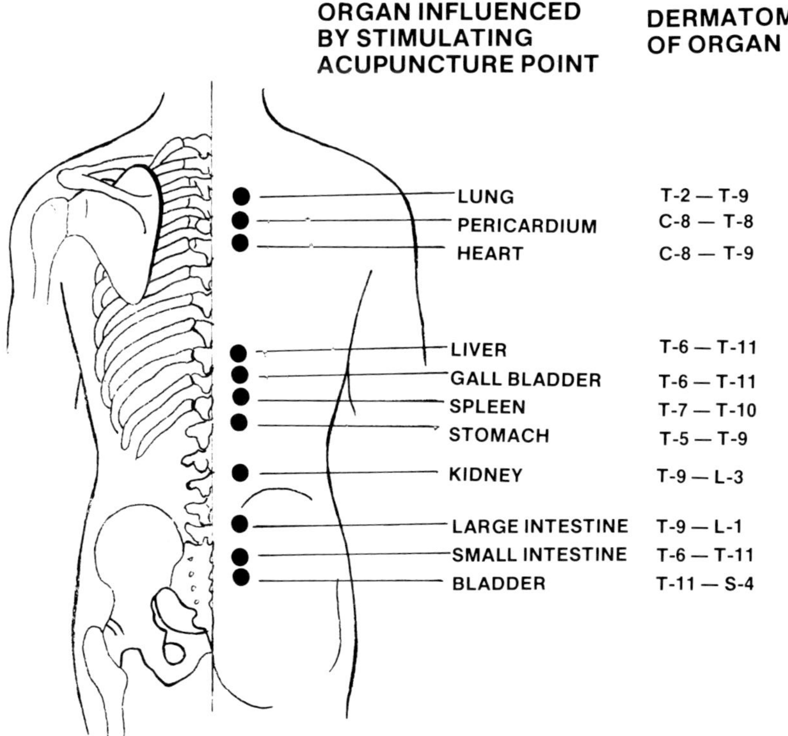

Figure 31. Correspondence between some para-vertebral acupuncture points and neurotome segments that innervate body organs.

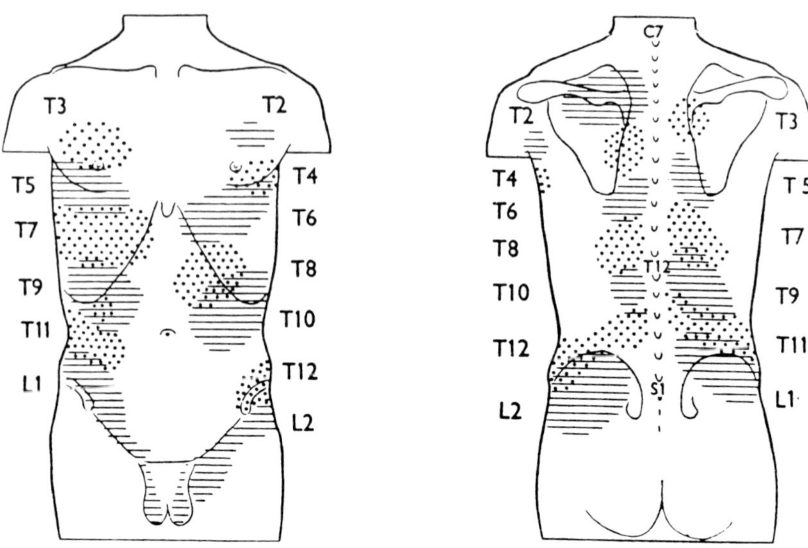

Figure 32. Distribution of pain on the body wall arising from stimulation of interspinous ligaments. A presumed mechanism for referral of pain from organ dysfunction within the same neurotome. From Kellgren, J.K.: On the distribution of pain arising from deep somatic structures with charts of segmental pain areas. *Clinical Science*, 1939-42, 4:35-36.

On the face, head and neck areas the same principles may be followed. The Chinese have long used the daily massage of points around the orbit for the promotion of good vision and the treatment of ocular problems. The facial point, Ying hsiang (LI-20), has a clinically demonstrated effect upon the mucous linings of the nasal cavity and has, thus, been useful for the relief of sinus congestion. Its translation "welcome fragrance" speaks directly of its efficacy. Several points around the external ear are felt to have a reflex action, probably vascular, that may produce some relief from VIIIth nerve afflictions.

Autonomic effects may be achieved by stimulation not only of the corresponding posterior rami but also by reflex action of more distant peripheral points (42). It has been shown by Matsumoto (12) that stimulation of ST-36 can induce peristalsis in post-surgical atony of the gut, both in rabbits and in man. Omura (83), has demonstrated that the stimulation of many acupuncture points can produce effects upon microcirculation. There is initially vasoconstriction followed by a more prolonged vasodilitation.

Ear acupuncture illustrates well the use of cutaneous points to affect visceral function. The ear is innervated by branches derived from the trigeminal nerve, facial nerve, glossopharyngeal nerve, vagus nerve, major auricular nerve and the minor occipital nerve. Of these the vagus is the most important (Figure 33). Points of low resistance were found in the rabbits ear in the area innervated by auricular branches of the vagus nerve (105). Probably the major basis for the effectiveness of ear acupuncture is the fact that the concha of the ear is the only place on the surface of the body where one can easily stimulate fibers of the vagus nerve (Nerve of Arnold). This nerve reaches many of the major viscera of the body and therefore represents a parasympathetic homeostatic regulatory mechanism.

It thus appears evident that referred pain and acupuncture share the same pathways within a single neurotome with the skin (dermatome) at one end and the internal organ (splanchnotome) at the other. Thus when disturbance occurs in an organ, pain can be referred to a corresponding skin area. Acupuncture at this point of maximal tenderness can induce a cutaneo-visceral reflex attenuating the referred pain and the visceral disturbance (89).

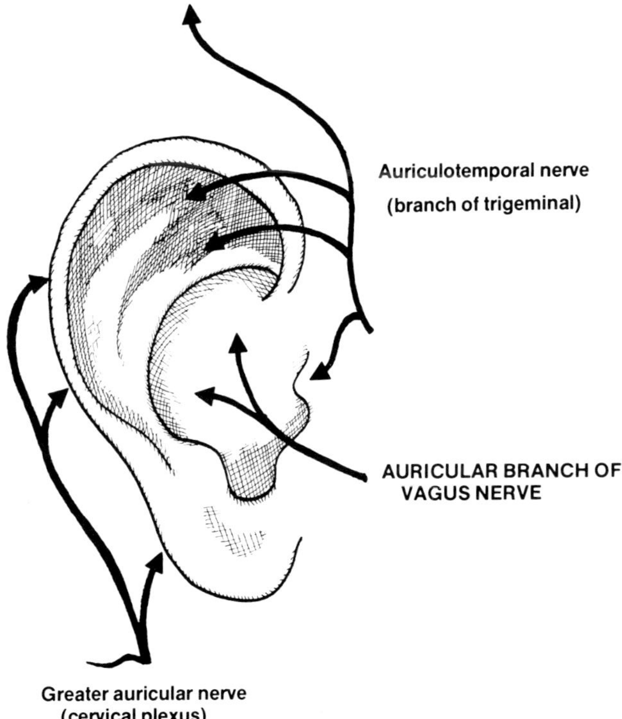

Figure 33. Innervation of the ear.

D. TRIGGER POINTS AND REFERENCE AREAS ON PAIN

At times it may be appropriate to select points for acupuncture stimulation according to the localization of trigger point reflex pain areas in the manner of techniques elucidated by Travell beginning in 1942 (106,107,108). She described small hypersensitive loci in the myofascial structures that when stimulated, touched or probed give rise to a larger area of pain in an adjacent or distant reference area. She noted that such trigger points were more or less constant in location from one person to another. It will be seen in the accompanying illustrations adapted from her work (Figure 34, a-d) that many of the designated trigger spots are identical or similar in location to some acupuncture points. This concordance of acupuncture points and trigger points has been reported to be as high as 71% (109). Other sensitive areas could well be the extra meridian "ouch" spots not infrequently used by acupuncturists in the treatment of pain.

Travell has postulated that some initial insult sets in motion a chain of events which is thus perpetuated by a vicious cycle of nerve impulses which have no further dependence upon afferent stimulation but rather are sustained by facilitation of the noxious stimuli in closed self reexciting chains of internuncial neurons in the central nervous system. The initial stimulus can be a direct trauma to the muscle, chronic muscular strain, chilling of fatigued muscles, acute myositis, arthritis, nerve root injury or visceral ischemia. Peripheral factors include fatigue, chronic infection and psychogenic stress. Electro-acupuncture can act by breaking up such reverberating neuronal circuits.

Protracted myofascial pain following pressure upon trigger points is thought to depend on a reflex pain cycle mediated by the trigger area. Travell reported both temporary and permanent relief from chronic myofascial pain by dry needling of these trigger areas. It is of interest that in some of the trigger/reflex areas she observed that the symptom pattern could be of a complex nature rather than simple pain. Thus, a trigger spot in the sterno-cleido-mastoid muscle, for example, was described as producing dizziness, imbalance, and headaches, with at times nausea, vomiting and tinnitus. She also demonstrated the relief of headaches, breast pain, cardiac pain and other symptoms by needle stimulation of appropriate cutaneous reference zones for such visceral disturbance.

→

Figure 34 a—d. Pain pattern and trigger areas. From Travell, J., and Rinzler, S.H.: The myofascial genesis of pain. Scientific Exhibit shown at Annual Session of American Medical Association Mtg., Atlantic City, 1951. *Postgrad. Med.*, 2:425-434, 1952.

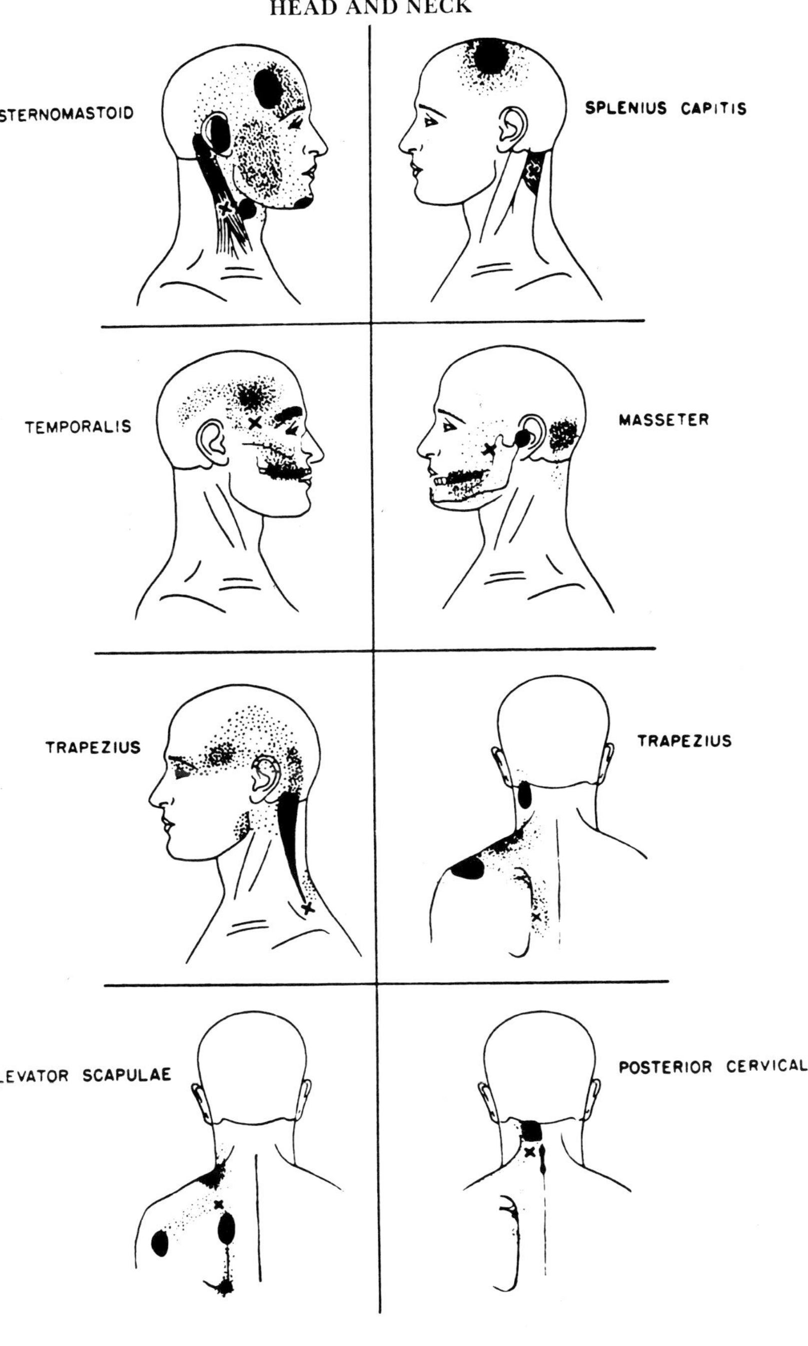
HEAD AND NECK
STERNOMASTOID
SPLENIUS CAPITIS
TEMPORALIS
MASSETER
TRAPEZIUS
TRAPEZIUS
LEVATOR SCAPULAE
POSTERIOR CERVICAL
PAIN PATTERN
TRIGGER AREA X

Figure 34 A.

SHOULDER AND ARM

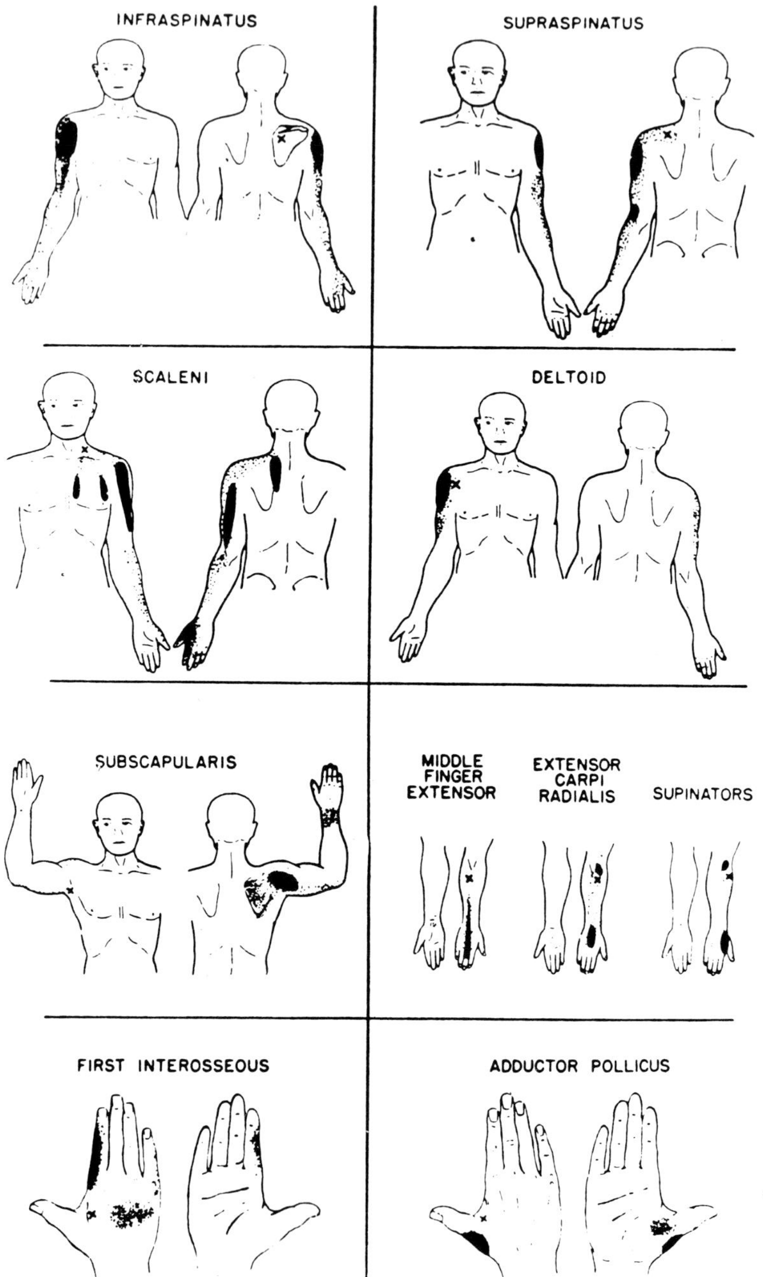

Figure 34 B.

CHEST AND BACK

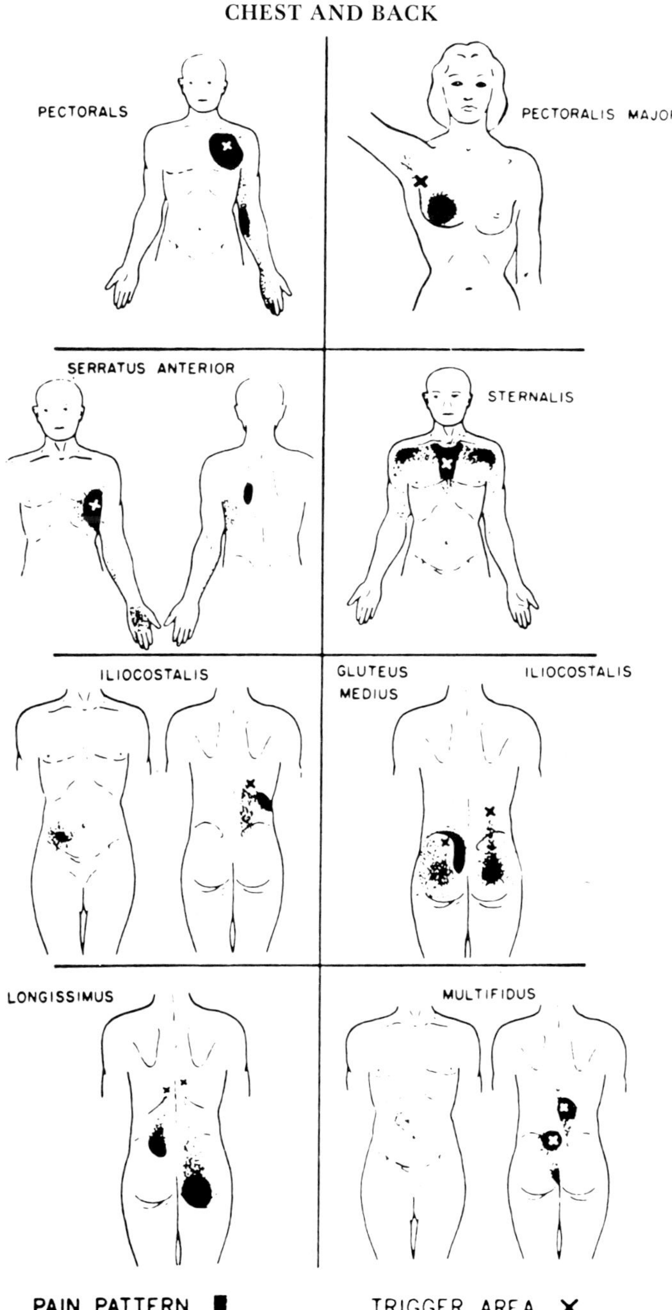

Figure 34 C.

LOWER EXTREMITY

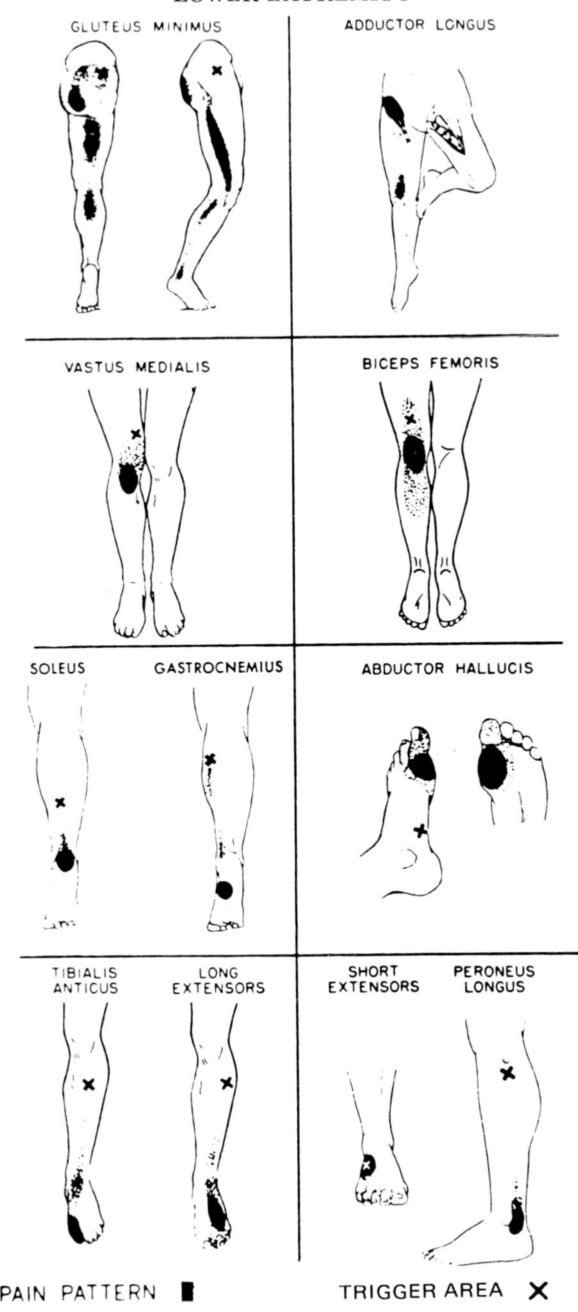

Figure 34 D.

E. SUMMARY—PROCEDURE

From the above discussion of motor points, viscero-cutaneous reflexes and trigger points, it can be seen that there are several choices of point selection for electro-acupuncture stimulation. Any of these methods of point selection may be utilized for sequential treatment sessions or selection of several points from each method might be used during a single treatment session. The complex interacting pathways of the central nervous system permit a single point of stimulation to be active in several ways and, as well, for the stimulation of several selected points to effect relief in a single area or organ system.

Our procedure is to initially search for trigger points. When such a point or points are found an acupuncture needle is inserted directly and deeply into the muscle tissue in the center of the point. If finger pressure on the point has produced referred pain to another area that area is also so treated.

Should trigger points not be present needles are inserted into motor points of the afflicted area as near as possible to the point of pain. As we customarily use a stimulator with four pairs of leads we use eight acupuncture needles. With electrical stimulation two needles are required for each stimulating circuit. We usually place an even number of needles—2,4,6 or 8—around the area of pain. It is, however, not necessary that the needles be connected in any particular fashion. For any pair of leads the needles may be several feet apart, in different parts of the body or even on different limbs.

If the affected area does not require or permit the insertion of all eight needles we may then place some of the needles in those points located approximately one and one half inches lateral to the spine. The point selected then is close to the exit of the nerve root of the neurotome corresponding to the affected area. If we cannot find a trigger spot or have found the use of trigger spots and/or motor points to be relatively ineffective, we may use only these para-spinal, neurotome (BL) points. Thus, depending upon the progress of the patient, we may from treatment-to-treatment vary our selection of the points to be used.

In the treatment of conditions other than pain we use primarily stimulation of the neurotome corresponding to the organ or organ system involved—again para-spinal points. For psychosomatic conditions and anxiety we prefer to use two needles, one in the concha of each ear.

All electrical stimuli are at low frequencies, 2-5 Hertz and with initial adjustment to a level where the patient can just feel the stimulus comfortably or, if in or near a motor point, to an intensity that will cause the needle to vibrate. We do not later increase the current even though the patient may report an adaptation so that the current pulses are no longer perceptable. Thus throughout the treatment the volume control is not changed. The duration of the stimulation is from 15-20 minutes.

F. SELECTION OF ACUPUNCTURE POINTS BY FORMULA

Most acupuncture today is taught and performed on the basis of formulae. There are certain sets of points recommended for use with each specific illness or symptom. A major difficulty with this approach lies in the fact that such formulae have been only empirically determined and their validity as yet untested by scientific means. As one pursues the published literature on acupuncture it becomes quickly evident that there is little agreement on the formulae to be used for most major illnesses. To date, there has been no acceptable research comparing these formulations either as to their validity or reliability.

The reasons for such widespread use of "acupuncture by formulae" are several: *First*, traditional acupuncture point selection is based upon complicated metaphysical theories for balancing an hypothesized disruption of yin/yang energy as detected by pulse diagnosis. Although such a fanciful ritual may have been acceptable in pre-scientific times, with increasing knowledge of anatomy and physiology point selection in this manner is scientifically untenable. Those who remain loyal to such traditional metaphysical beliefs use the excuse that "only a few master acupuncturists are capable of using pulse diagnosis" and, hence, acupuncturists of lesser skill must rely upon formulae.

Second, according to the teachings of the Nei Ching (110), acupuncture performed in accordance with the traditional theoretical concepts was of value primarily for the prevention of illness and should therefore, be used only before any serious symptoms of disease become manifest. When signs of major illness were obvious, it was traditionally taught that the energy within the meridians at that time exhibited such a state of fluctuating imbalance that accurate pulse diagnosis was impossible and treatment must begin with needle placement designated by formulae.

Third, with the recent blending of Western medicine and traditional techniques of acupuncture, the diagnosis of disease became increasingly a matter for laboratory methods and Western physical diagnostic techniques. Illnesses are now given diagnostic labels acceptable to international medical terminology. Thus, energy balancing receives much less attention and needle placement on meridian points has been increasingly matched to formulae designated as specifically effective for each type of illness as ascertained by Western diagnosis.

The problem then is that of selecting "which formula for which disease?" It becomes evident from even a preliminary scan of the books on acupuncture that many "experts" have many different sets of points for the same illness. Acupuncture was long an unwritten art, teaching passed from father to son with many secret formulations. Master acupuncturists have also been renowned for their special techniques and "miracle cures." Thus, the use of acupuncture by formulae has a long history. Empirically, some of these formulae may have been effective simply because the designated points selected happened to lie over physiologically active areas such as motor points or along major nerve trunks. Despite its many contradictions the method is universally used and thus perhaps worthy of note at this time of flux from the traditional to a more scientifically based procedure. The use of set formulae may be useful for the beginning practitioner of acupuncture who, when confronted by the first patients, puzzles over optimal needle placement. As patients come in with similar complaints there is a tendency to use a similar array of needles. Thus, with experience, there is developed one's own set of preferred formulae. Even these, however, will be varied from patient-to-patient and from treatment to treatment to meet the slight but significant differences in site of pain, body asymetries and the like.

In Table V with accompanying diagrams we list a few formulae from leading books on the subject. We have attempted to designate points upon which there was some agreement among several authors and, as far as possible, use those points with physiological rationale.

Although some authorities have listed as many as 20 points for a single condition, we have tried to limit our recommendations to a small number of points for each formula with the suggestion that other regionally appropriate points be added as the variations in location, character and intensity of symptoms are found to vary from patient-to-patient. As experience is gained from the successful treatment of patients one will feel confident using a smaller rather than a large number of needles. It is reported in traditional Chinese acupuncture that the master acupuncturist can cure with "but a single, well placed needle."

TABLE V
Acupuncture Point Formulae for the Treatment of Selected Conditions

WRIST AND HAND PAIN

LI-4
LI-11
HE-7
LU-7

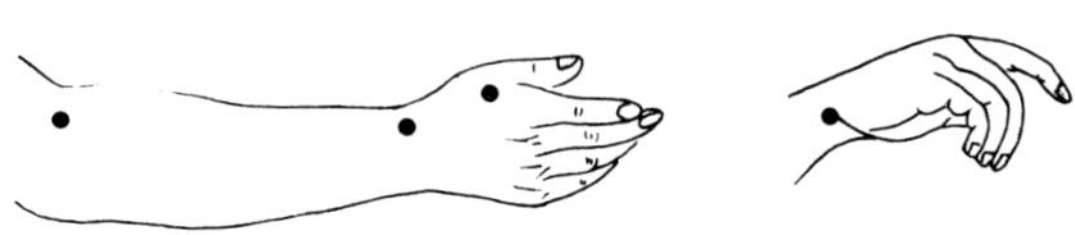

HIP AND LEG PAIN

GB-30
GB-31
GB-34
BL-50
BL-51

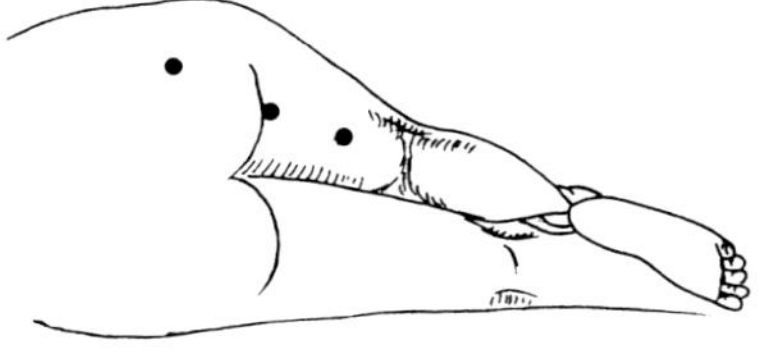

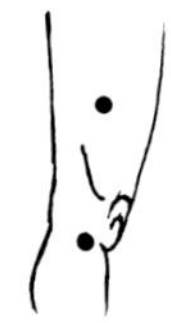

SCIATICA

GB-30
BL-54
BL-25
BL-57
BL-60
BL-23
BL-51

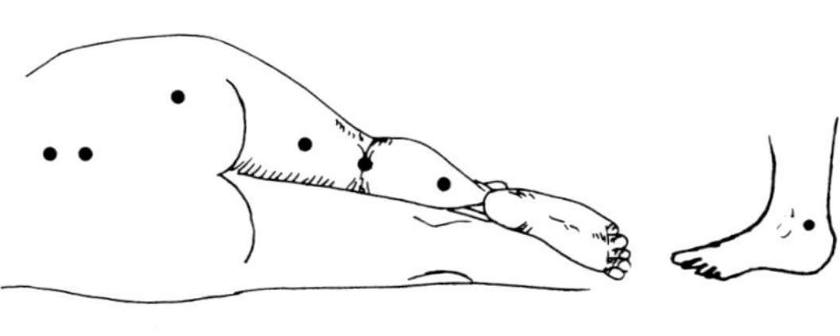

KNEE PAIN

GB-34
SP-10
BL-54
ST-36
ST-32

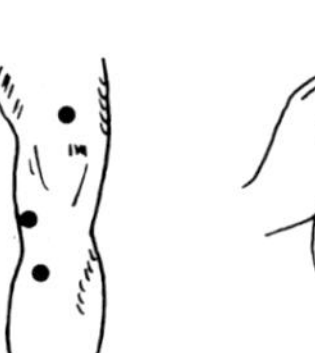

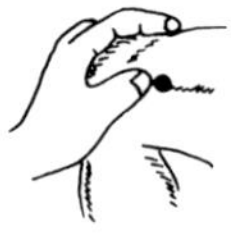

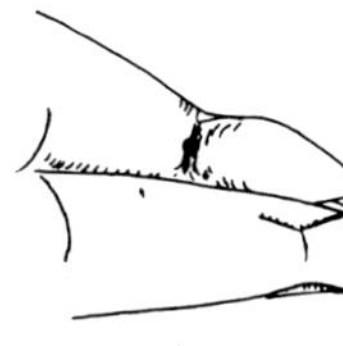

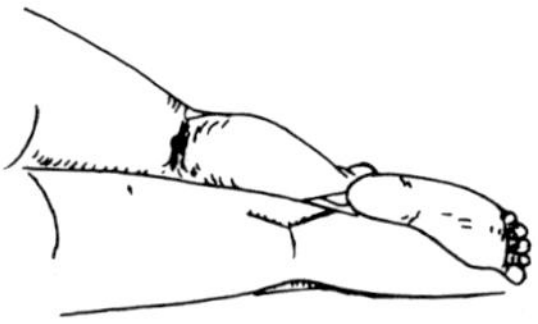

TABLE V (Cont.)

ANKLE AND FOOT PAIN

BL-60
KI-3
ST-44
LV-3

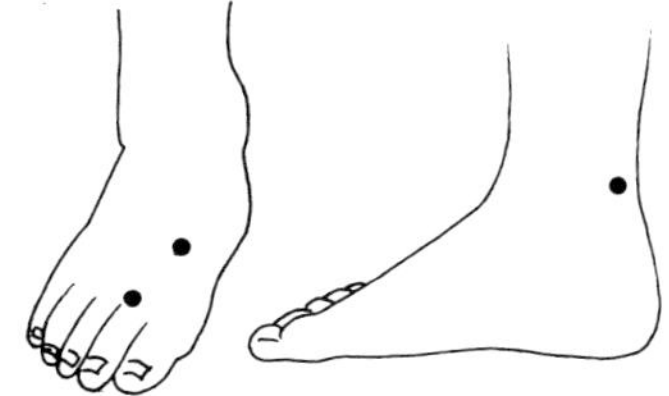

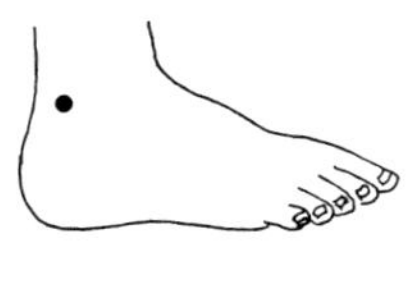

LOW BACK PAIN

INTERCOSTAL NEURALGIA

POST-HERPETIC NEURALGIA

PARAVERTEBRAL POINTS
AT LEVEL OF LESION

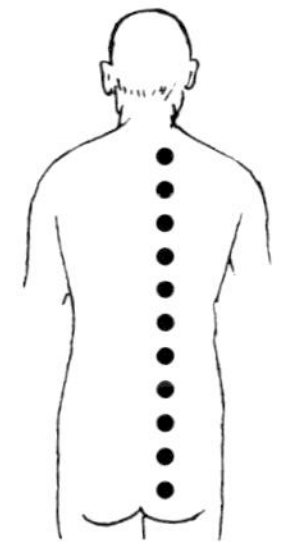

GASTRALGIA

CV-12
BL-21
ST-36
BL-18
LI-4
CV-3
CONCHA OF EAR

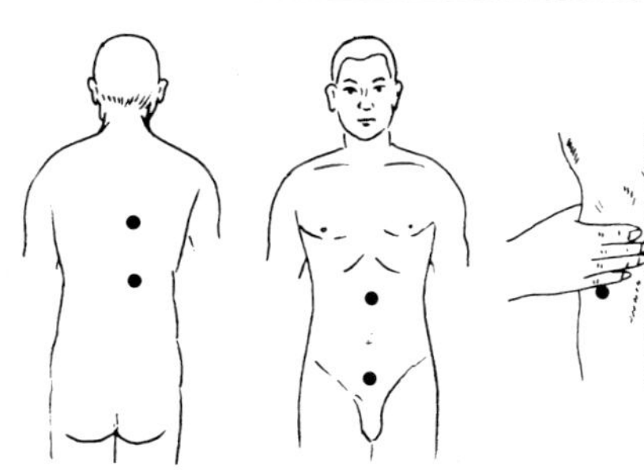

HEMIPLEGIA

LI-16
TH-5
LI-11
LI-4

GB-30
GB-31
GB-34
ST-36
SP-6

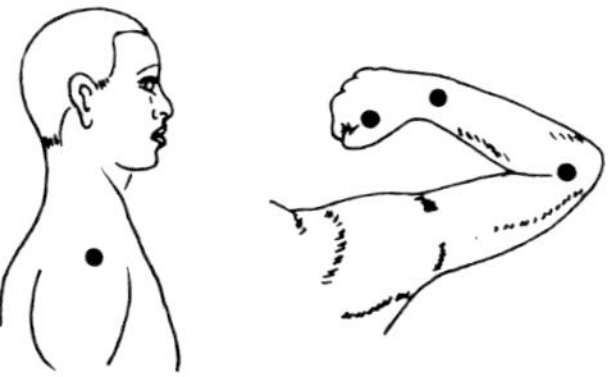

UPPER LIMB

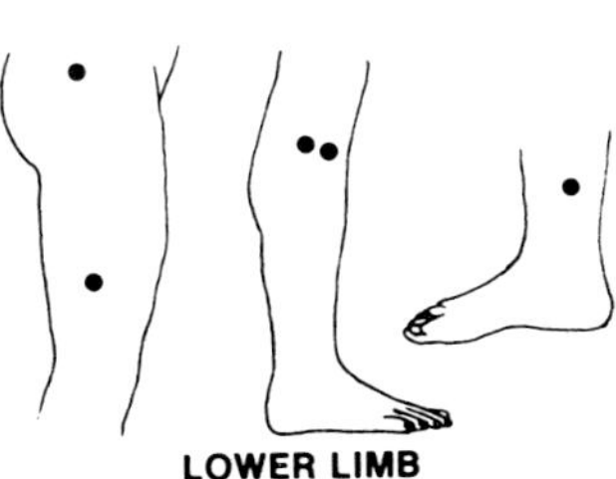

LOWER LIMB

TABLE V (Cont.)

TEMPERO-MANDIBULAR JOINT PAIN

LI-4
TH-21
SI-19

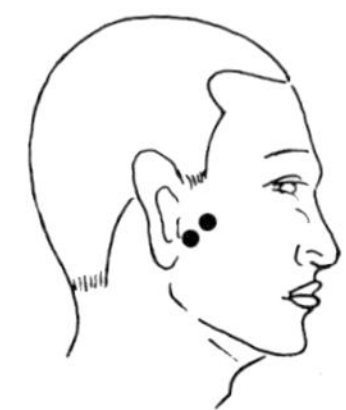
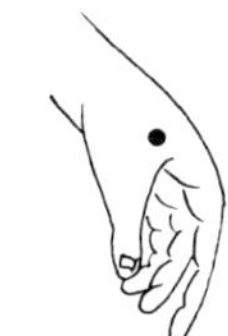

NECK PAIN

GB-20
GB-21
LI-4
TH-14

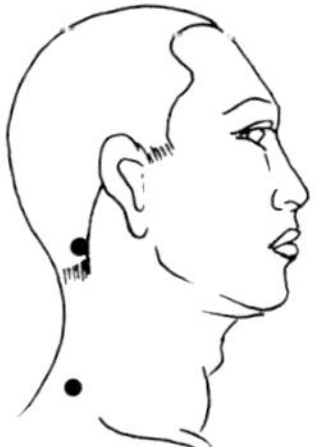
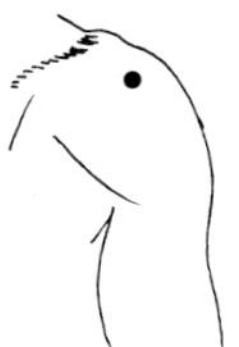
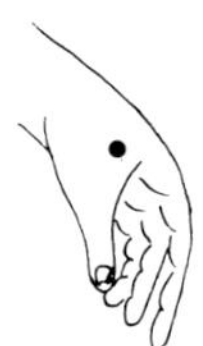

SHOULDER PAIN

LI-14
LI-16
TH-14
GB-21
LI-11
SP-20

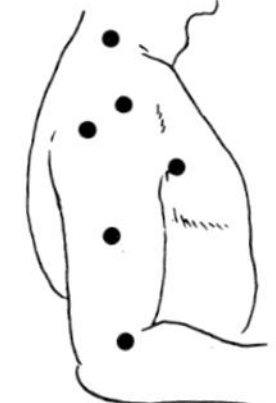
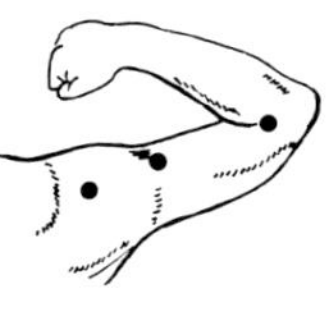

ELBOW PAIN

LI-11
TH-10
LI-4

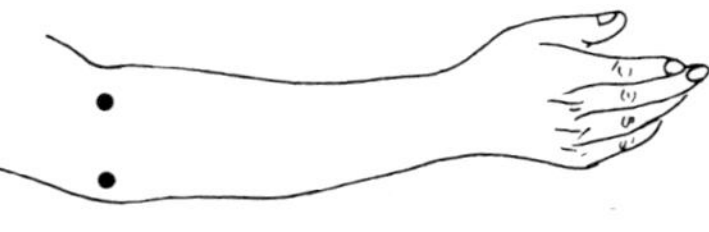
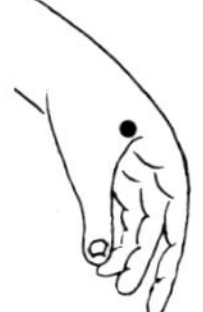

TABLE V (Cont.)

RHINITIS AND SINUSITIS

GB-20
LI-4
LI-20
BL-2

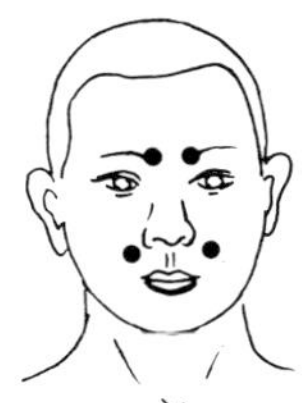
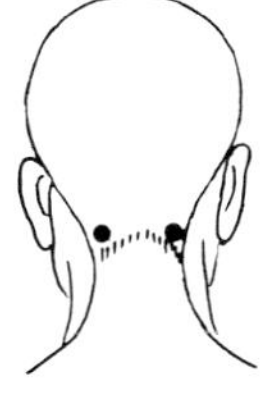
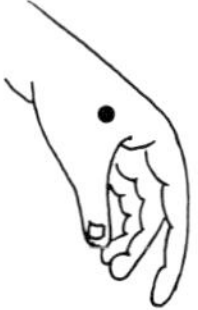

NERVE DEAFNESS
TINNITUS-VERTIGO

ST-7
TH-21
SI-19
TH-17
GB-20

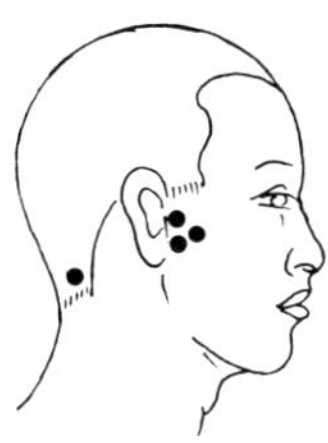
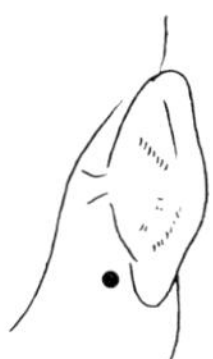

ANXIETY
ASTHMA
HYPERTENSION

CONCHA OF EAR

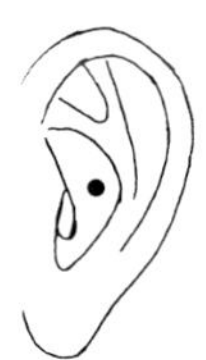

DEPRESSION

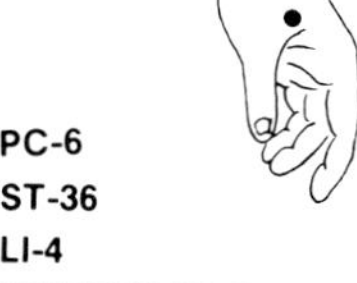
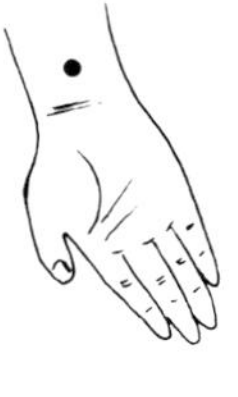
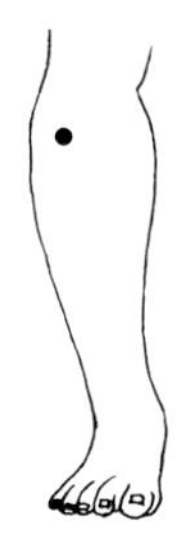
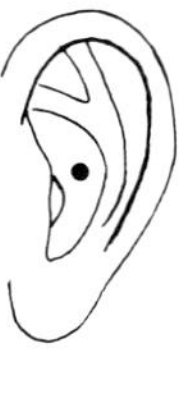

PC-6
ST-36
LI-4
CONCHA OF EAR

TABLE V (Cont.)

TOOTHACHE

LI-4
ST-7
ST-6
ST-4
ST-5

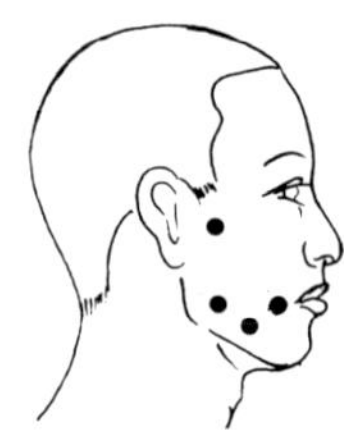
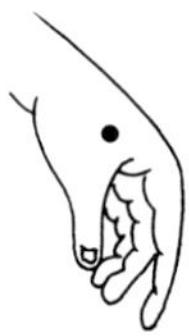

HEADACHE

GB-20
LI-4
EM-1
GV-20
GV-15

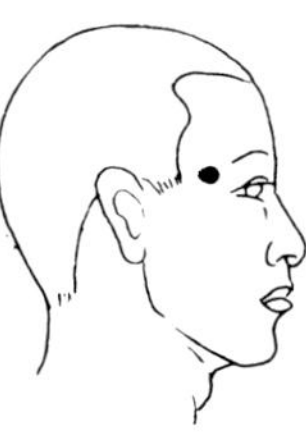
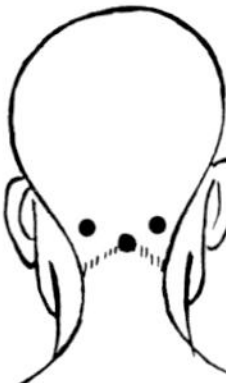
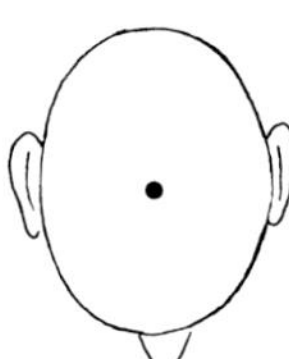
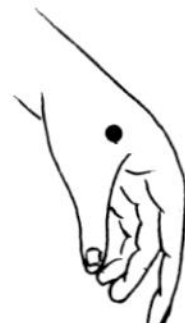

FACIAL PALSY

BL-2
ST-4
LI-4
ST-7

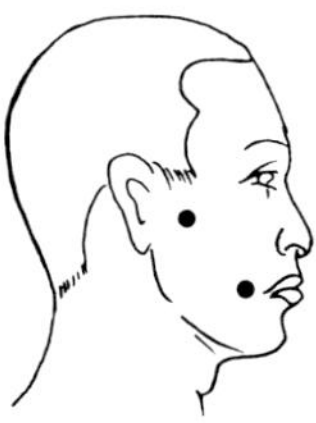
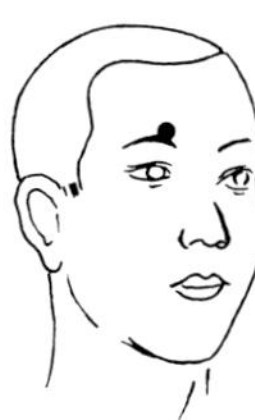
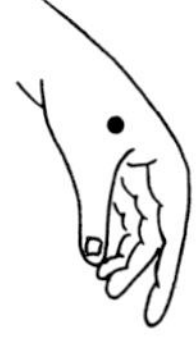

TABLE V (Cont.)

MENSTRUAL DYSFUNCTION

SP-6
SP-10
CV-3
CV-6

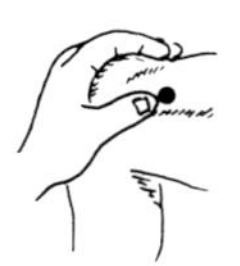
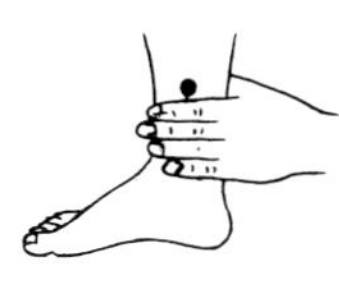
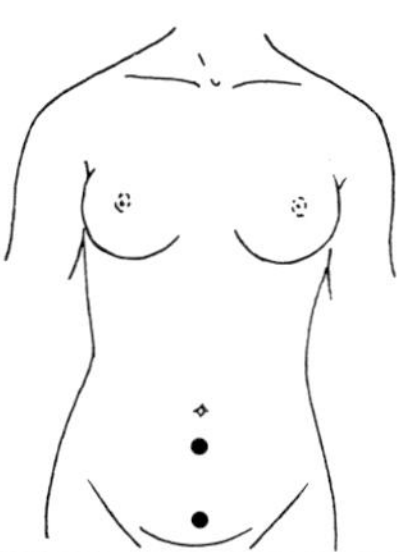

IMPOTENCE

BL-23
BL-50
SP-6
CV-3
ST-36
CONCHA OF EAR

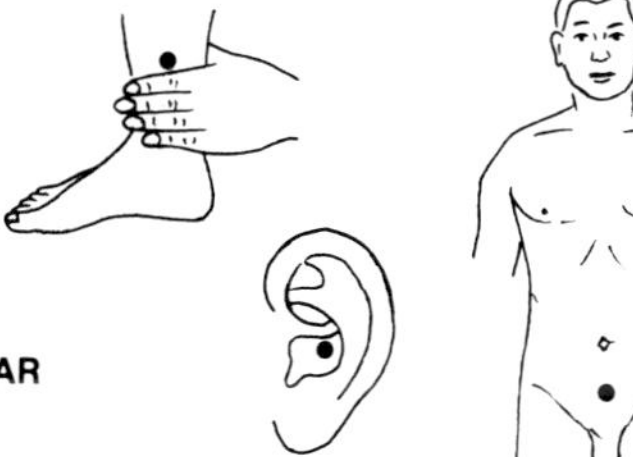
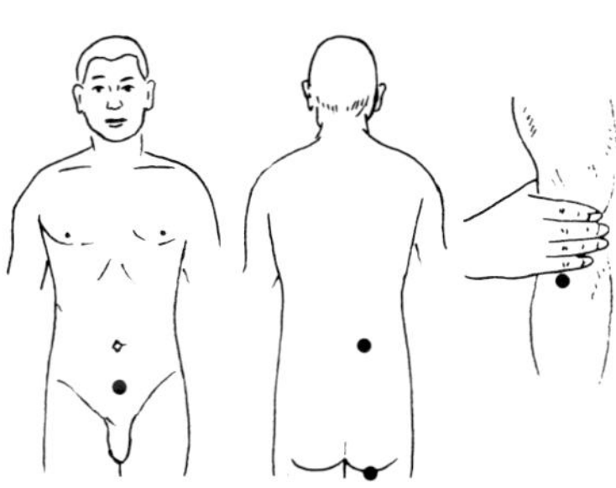

TRIGEMINAL NEURALGIA

TH-21
BL-2 OPHTHALMIC
EM-1

LI-20
GV-26
LI-4 MAXILLARY
ST-1

ST-7
ST-6 MANDIBULAR
ST-4
SI-19

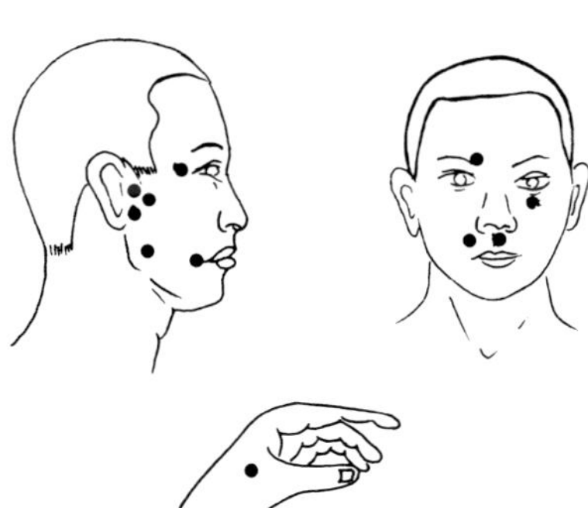

VI

NEEDLING TECHNIQUES

Acupuncture needles are fine wires, they bend easily and do not always readily pierce the skin. Many patients, recalling childhood immunization "shots" think of needles with great apprehension. On very rare occasions acupuncture needles have punctured intestines and collapsed lungs. Improper sterilization has resulted in bacterial infection and viral hepatitis. With proper technique all of the above can be avoided. The rules given here are simple and should become routine.

1. Patient Position

We have found lying down on the side with the affected side up, supine or prone as the best positions. For needle placement in the head, neck, shoulders, chest or extremities, the patient may be seated. As some patients are fearful of "needles," a resting position may avoid the occasional fainting that can occur, particularly during the first few treatments.

2. *Needles*

Needles come in a variety of types, gauges and lengths. "Hao" needles, (Figure 35), most commonly used are obtainable in gauge numbers 26-(0.45mm), 28-(0.38mm), 30-(0.32mm) and 32-(0.26mm). Heavy needles are more painful. Fine needles are easily bent—28-30 gauge are the most popular.

Needles vary in length. Common sizes include 0.5, 1.0, 1.5, 2.0, 2.5, 3 and 5 inches in length. The length selected depends upon the site for penetration. We have found 1.5 inch needles to be generally useful with 0.5 preferable about the face and 2.5 and 3.0 useful for the gluteal areas or in heavily muscled patients.

Needles should be sterilized, preferably in the autoclave like surgical instruments. They may be kept sharp with sandpaper or an emery stone. If the patient has a history of viral hepatitis, the needles should be discarded or the same set should be used throughout the remainder of that patient's treatments.

In China, other types of needles are available. These are more of historical rather than practical use. The triple edge wedge shaped needles are used for bleeding and the plum, 5 and 7 star pronged needles or a hammer type needle used for tapping on the skin of infants for determatological conditions and local areas of edema. Fine, intradermal needles are inserted and left in the skin for extended periods of time. These are usually silver and may be in the shape of a thumbtack. They

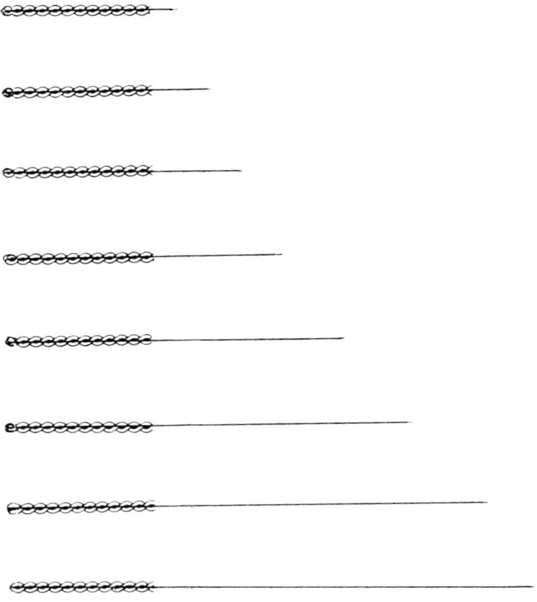

Figure 35. Acupuncture needles.

are called "press needles" and are used for auriculotherapy. Placement of catgut sutures is used in China. These are threaded through acupuncture points and left in position for long periods of time.

3. *Needle Insertion*

There is very little pain associated with proper needle technique. The more rapid the insertion the better. The fingers should be clean and the skin cleansed with alcohol prior to needle insertion. The needle is held by the lower stem section and in between the thumb and index finger of the right hand, exposing about 2mm of the needle (Figure 36). With a quick thrust this is pushed through the skin at the acupuncture point. The hand then moves to the needle handle and with a twirling motion the needle is drilled into the subcutaneous tissue. With two handed techniques the left hand holds the needle against the skin while the right hand drills. Or, the fingernail of the left index finger can push against the acupuncture point while the needle is directed into the point by the right thumb and forefinger. This is useful in areas about the head and face. In such areas, too, it may be useful to pinch the skin and place the needle between the two fingers that are holding the skin.

The depth of insertion must be governed by the size of the muscle mass

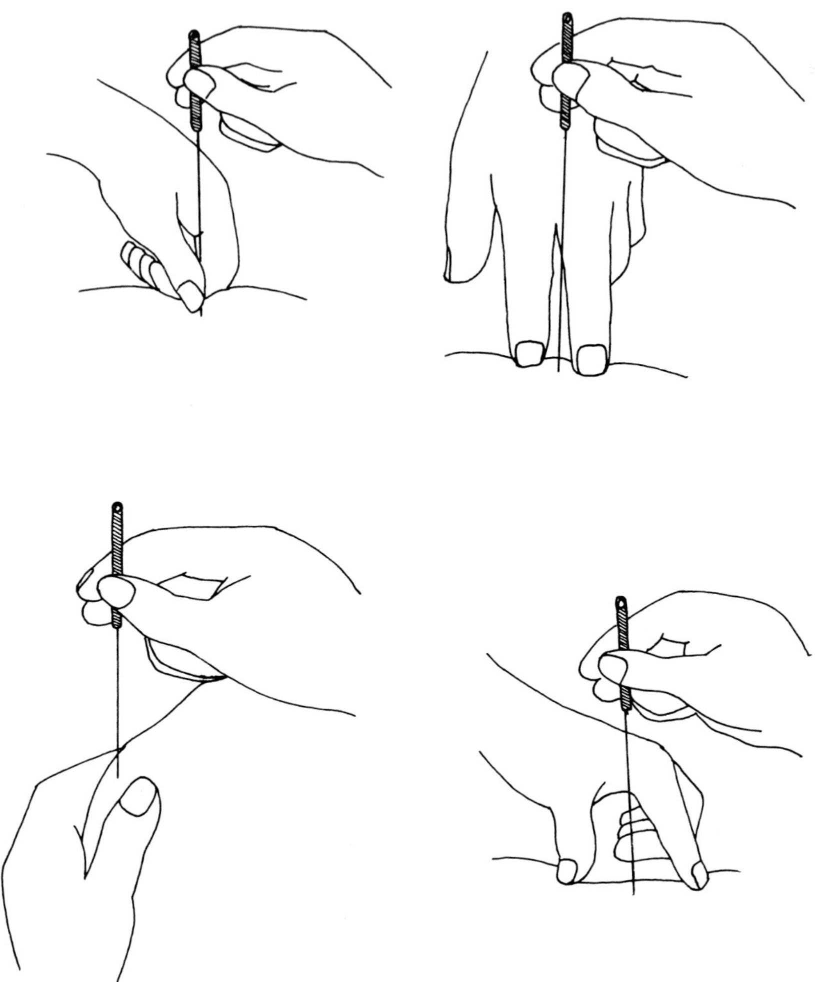

Figure 36. Methods of needle insertion.

in the area being stimulated. It is not possible to give a figure for safe depth of insertion at each point as there is so much variation from one person to another. A sound knowledge of anatomy is therefore necessary for the practice of acupuncture. Where there is doubt about muscle mass a shallow penetration is preferable. Wherever possible the needle should penetrate to the motor point although it often appears, especially with electrical stimulation, that a good effect can be obtained with superficial insertion.

Needles should usually be inserted vertically, at 90 degrees perpendicular to the skin for the most accurate access to the motor point in the underlying tissue. In order to bypass important bones, organs, etc., a 45 degree angle may be used. For many points about the face and head needles are inserted along under the skin at about a 15 degree angle.

The very fine needles used by the Japanese are inserted through a hollow metal tube (a length of a plastic soda straw cut to proper size may be used as a disposable tube). The tube should be 2mm shorter than the needle (Figure 37). The tube is pressed over the acupuncture point until the patient feels only the pressure. A quick tap or snap of the finger with the fingernail against the top of the needle pushes the needle painlessly through the skin. After penetration, the tube is removed and the needle is painlessly drilled to the proper depth. When properly used these needles produce less pain and are particularly useful about the face. They do require more time for insertion.

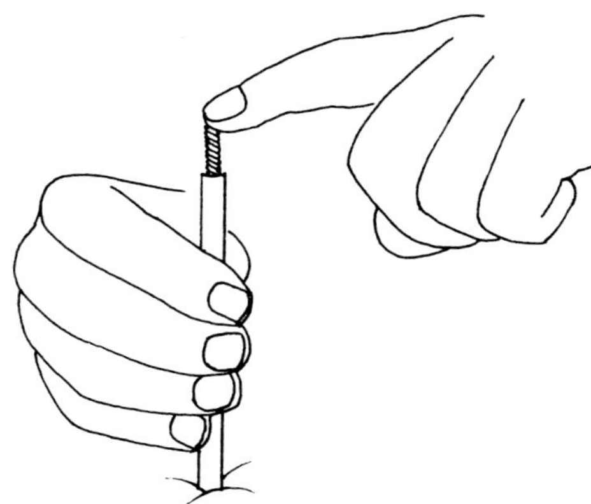

Figure 37. Hollow tube method of inserting fine Japanese acupuncture needles.

*4. Needle Sensation**

This sensation occurs when the needle point is at or near the neurovascular hilus (motor point). It is elicited by moving or twirling the needle. It is usually described by the patient as a dull ache, drawing sensation, heat or throbbing. This awareness of the needle is not described as painful. It results from the stimulation of the receptors of the muscles, nerves, proprioceptors, mechanoreceptors, nociceptors, autonomic fibers, etc. This sensation occurs within seconds of insertion. It is abolished by local anesthetics at the motor point, but not by local anesthetic to the skin.

*Called "teh chi" in Chinese acupuncture.

5. Needle Grasp

Withdrawal of the needle may be impaired by a superficial gripping related to local contraction of the elastic connective tissue of the skin. A deeper grasping, which can result in a bent needle may occur at motor points within the muscle layers. This has been explained as a "gamma loop" phenomenon and more frequently occurs with some motor or sensory lesions which sensitize the annulospiral endings and flower spray endings around the intra-fusal fibers. When such afferent endings are hypersensitive, the needle puncture elicits a stimulus that, in turn, causes an effector response from the gamma fibers of the ventral horn with strong contractions of the muscle bulk. This may be thought of as a decompensation of the automatic gain-control mechanism of the muscle fibers. (111)

6. Needle Withdrawal

When the treatment is finished a cotton ball may be placed firmly over the acupuncture point as the needle is withdrawn. Continued firm pressure or a light massage can halt any small bleeding that may rarely occur and could leave a temporary subcutaneous discoloration. It is well to alert patients to this occurence, as they may later become apprehensive over the appearance of what appears to be a bruise. Should some secondary lymph or blood escape into the tissues subcutaneously a hot compress can hasten absorption.

7. Stimulation

For centuries needles were simply inserted into acupuncture points and left for varying periods of time. If a needle sensation was elicited, a brief period of a minute or two was felt to be sufficient for treatment. Twirling of the needles produced additional stimulation. This was accomplished by the finger and thumb of the right hand rotating the shaft of the needle in a rapid alternating clockwise and counterclockwise motion while at the same time exerting a push-pull movement. Bilateral stimulation, that is with a symmetrical placement of two needles, is often used when inner organs are involved or with central pain as with headache, gastric problems, etc.

In recent years acupuncturists have found that electrical stimulation is superior and certainly easier to apply than methods of manual manipulation. Our studies (36), have shown electrical stimulation to be approximately 100% more effective than simple needle placement. Because electro-acupuncture produces a stronger stimulation it is often best to reserve it for the second and subsequent sessions, especially in patients who are initially apprehensive. With electrical stimulation some benefit may be achieved even if a needle is not precisely located due to the spread of current through the tissues. When visible muscle fasciculation occurs the needle is within or near a motor point.

The stimulator is attached to the needles by small clips. The paired wires are usually attached to needles that are nearby each other although no definite rules have been developed for such selection. The number of needles stimulated depends upon the number of lead jacks in the electric stimulator, usually three or four, thus six or eight needles can be connected. Figure 38 shows a stimulator of Chinese manufacture that permits stimulation of several needles with controls for varying Hertz and intensity.

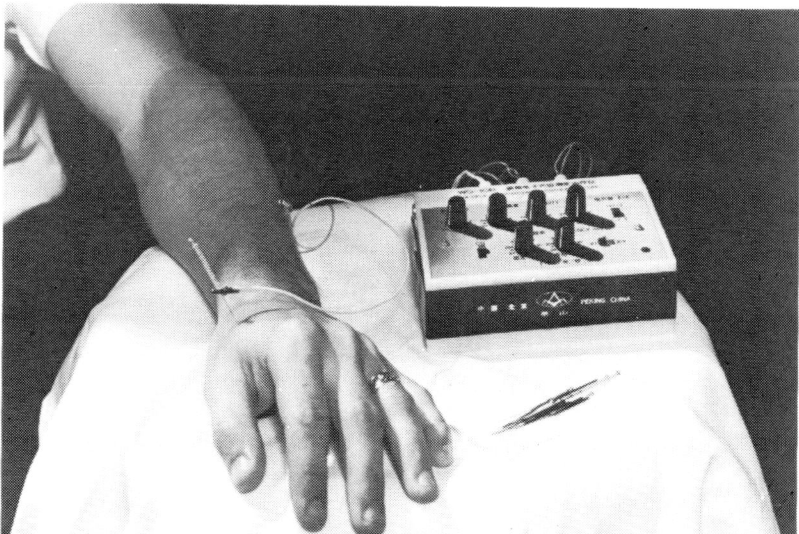

Figure 38. Typical electronic acupuncture stimulator of Chinese manufacture.

A great deal of investigation remains to be done to ascertain the ideal parameters of stimulation for different types of application. Currently, it is felt that useful stimulation can occur with currents reported to vary from 0.5 to 50 milliamps. Voltages are from 0.3 to 9 volts usually produced by a 9 volt dry cell source. The wave forms vary but are customarily square waves or waves of exponentially rising or falling form, from 0.1 to 0.3 milliseconds duration and occuring in trains. These thus are pulsating DC potentials.

Pulses from 1 Hz to 1000 Hz have been used. Some workers feel that slow pulsations (1-10) Hz are best for acute pain and fast (80-120) Hz for chronic pain. This belief is not universally held. Bowsher (112), has commented on the inability of neurons of the reticular formation to respond to peripheral stimulation at frequencies above 3 Hz. We customarily use slow pulses for the treatment of all painful conditions. Some have reported relief of recurrent pain by 20 minutes of stimulation at 2-3 Hz with such relief lasting from 1-2 and 2½ days from a single session. There is speculation that the serotonergic system of pain modulation is activated by high frequency electro-acupuncture while the endorphinergic system responds to low frequency electro-acupuncture.

We usually stimulate from 15-30 minutes at each session. Although there is little data in the scientific literature to support any specific amount of stimulation, most reports indicate that improvement will occur within 6-8 treatments. Occasionally patients will improve after only one or two treatments while others require many more. Occasionally patients get no therapeutic response until after 10-12 treatments. Initially, some patients are treated 2-3 times a week, later one treatment a week is sufficient. In patients with severe pain, treatment may be given two times a day, five days a week. In other patients, with chronic arthritis for example, it has been useful after an initial course to continue on a one-time-a-month schedule. We have found such a schedule may prevent relapse. Other patients obtain complete relief after six or eight treatments and do not require any more. Pain relief is usually cummulative with successive treatments although here, too, the course of recovery may be irregular. If we find no relief in eight to ten treatments we usually feel that, at least in our hands, acupuncture is not an appropriate modality for that patient.

The duration of relief from a single treatment varies greatly. Vierck, *et al.* (113), found in monkeys that the suppression of pain from a single treatment could last up to 70 hours but that the pain threshold showed major fluctuation during that time. While we sometimes see immediate relief it seems, with chronic pain, more likely that the greatest relief may appear one or two days after the treatment. On occasion the pain seems to increase for a few hours following the treatment before a longer period of abatement.

The level of stimulation required varies from patient-to-patient and for the same patient from day-to-day. The patient should feel the stimulation and may have some muscle fibrillation. The current is adequate when either of the above occurs. The level of stimulation should not produce discomfort during the treatment. Once we have adjusted the stimulation to a comfortable level we do not again change the setting but rather maintain that level of stimulation throughout the duration of the treatment. Often the patient will state that the stimulus is no longer felt. This is simply body accomodation, with the level of stimulation remaining the same. In susceptible individuals reddening of the skin can occur with simple placement of the needle. It is more often seen with electro-acupuncture stimulation. With careful adjustment of the current, skin burns are never seen. One theoretical grounds and because of the possible danger of inducing cardiac fibrillation, we avoid using electrostimulation around the precordium or in patients with implanted pacemakers.

8. *Patient Selection and Preparation*

We have treated patients of all ages with acupuncture. Although usually given in the physician's office, hospitals are increasingly tolerant of acupuncture procedures. Some insurance companies will reimburse, at least in part, for acupuncture and, particularly, if it is explained to them what it is, or described in other terms such as SENS (subcutaneous electrical nerve stimulation) or percutaneous electrical nerve stimulation.

There is no way to predict which patients will respond to electrical acupuncture stimulation. While it has been reported that hypnotizable subjects do better than non-hypnotizable subjects, this would seem to be a part of the generalization that positive suggestion added to any treatment will increase the yield. In our research and that of others, poorly hypnotizable subjects, human as well as animal, have done well with acupuncture (114). A positive attitude is said to be predictive but we have not found this universally true. We have successfully treated patients who were openly skeptical and who came to the office reluctantly at the urgence of a spouse. Less positive results are found in patients who have had previous surgery. Success on the first treatment has some positive predictive value.

Patients should be psychologically prepared by some discussion of the nature of acupuncture, the near absence of side effects, no great pain, etc. Patients should be placed in a comfortable position and cautioned against any gross movements of the body. The bladder should be emptied prior to treatment. The patient should have no alcohol or drugs active on the nervous system prior to treatment. Inquiries should be made concerning previous surgery in the area of treatment or near the passage of neurotomes that are selected for use.

9. *Side Effects and Complications*

a) Dizziness and Circulatory Shock (Fainting)

This is seen mostly in patients receiving acupuncture for the first time and is due to emotional stress, tension, fatigue, hunger or labile autonomic nervous system. We are wary of patients who are highly neurotic or who experience profuse sweating, tachycardia or those who have a weak thready pulse. We have such patients lie flat on the table and often in the initial treatment use very few needles and no electrical stimulation. Should the patient faint, lower the head or treat as if in shock and withdraw all of the needles. Strong stimulation of KI-1 on the sole of the foot may arouse the patient.

b) Severe Needle Grasp

This is due to muscle tension and can be overcome by relaxation of the patient or the application of a second needle at an angle adjacent to the impounded needle.

c) Bent Needle

Change the patient's position and withdraw the needle in the direction of the curve.

d) Broken Needle

We have never experienced this complication. It can be avoided by careful selection and discarding of eroded or defective needles. Removal by manipulation or the use of a hemostat would be the preferred method. Immediate surgery should rarely be necessary.

e) Hematoma

Upon removal of the needles each point should be carefully inspected for bleeding which may appear after the delay of a minute or two. Surface bleeding can be seen and controlled by pressure.

f) Infection

With autoclaved needles and clean techniques this should not occur. We have not had one occasion in several thousand patients. Transmission of viral hepatitis has been reported when the needle has been inadequately sterilized.

g) Organ Penetration

In the hands of unskilled practitioners with poor knowledge of human anatomy, penetration of organs, especially of the intestines, bladder, lungs, peritoneum and pleura, have been reported. Severe atalectasis has been reported on stimulation of shoulder points where the acupuncturist failed to recall that the apex of the left lung, especially in females, may be within reach of a two inch needle. Selection of needles should be appropriate to the depth of muscle in the area to be treated. Too shallow penetration is less effective and too deep penetration is dangerous.

10. Contraindications to Acupuncture

a) Patient inebriated, tense or perspiring freely.

b) Deep puncture over the abdomen or chest in the region of the lungs, heart, liver, spleen, kidney, intestines or bladder.

c) In pregnant women, especially points with lower lumbar or sacral outflow or on the abdomen below the umbilicus.

d) Avoid swollen or infected areas.

e) Avoid points in the epigastrium after a full meal.

f) Avoid cranial points near the fontanelles in children.

g) Avoid points on a woman's breast.

h) Avoid points on the testicle.

k) Care should be taken around large blood vessels as in the groin, near the aorta or vena cava.

VII

CLINICAL APPLICATION OF ACUPUNCTURE

The usefulness of acupuncture for pain relief is documented by numerous clinical reports and by theories of action that are both plausible for Western trained physicians and supported by theories concurrent with modern physiology and biochemistry. The use of acupuncture in psychosomatic illness, however, and for patients with emotional illnesses is less well documented but has been found useful by many physicians on an empirical basis. We have obtained some suprisingly good results in the treatment of a variety of conditions that have failed to respond to more traditional medical management.

In our own practice, as elsewhere, the major use of acupuncture is for the treatment of pain, both acute and chronic. Most common among our favorable responders are those who, treated on a once weekly basis, get only a small amount of pain relief after a treatment or two but then continue with a steady improvement week after week after week to a point where after 8-10 treatments, the pain is controlled for ever longer periods. At that point treatments can be given at bi-monthly and finally monthly or longer intervals. Many patients who receive almost complete relief require no additional treatments. Ours is an experience from private practice and we have not been able to conduct systematic follow up studies. We have, however, had numerous reports from new patients who tell us that they were referred to us by former patients of ours who have continued to do well over periods of months or years. We have had patients with arthritic or neuralgic conditions return to us with a pain that has returned, after asymptomatic periods of many months. They ask us to again give them the relief that they experienced with the original course of treatments and often this is accomplished with fewer treatments than were required the first time the patient was treated.

These clinical observations have served to strengthen our opinion that acupuncture acts in some "kindling-like" fashion that has a cumulative effect of dampening the activity in reverberating neuron pools. Such pools have a self-sustaining activity that tends to keep the pain threshold at a low level so that even the smallest increase in physical or emotional stress can produce suffering. With repeated stimuli from acupuncture treatments, one sees a steady, though sometimes uneven, remitting of such activity, a rise in pain threshold and, with the best of results a dropping out of such pain-producing activity. Undoubtedly these "pain memory" pools exist at several levels of the central nervous system including the cerebral cortex. We have successfully treated patients with phantom limb pain whose painful memories included the exact positioning of the limb at the time of an accident — a position which steadily corrected itself to a normal resting position with repeated acupuncture treatments.

Apart from musculo-fascial pain, pain of post-surgical nature, low back syndromes, athletic injuries and the like we have had considerable success with neuralgia, neuritis and headaches. We have treated cases of visceral pain, usually by vagal (ear) stimulation as well as posterior root stimulation at the level of visceral innervation. Results in the treatment of chronic nerve and muscle degenerative diseases, multiple sclerosis, stroke, nerve deafness and the like seem much more likely to be the result of some subjective improvement and probably have a larger placebo component. The fact that some such patients have, when undergoing acupuncture, reported an increased tempo in their rate of improvement has encouraged us to at least offer persons with this type of illness a trial of acupuncture treatment.

Acupuncture is also used for a variety of psychiatric conditions including depression, anxiety, insomnia, tension and nervousness. It has been suggested that the enkephalin and endorphin release which occurs with acupuncture involves as well the release of growth hormones and prolactin (117, 118, 119, 120). This hormonal release gives some credence to the use of acupuncture in such a wide range of conditions. We also feel that stimulation of the concha of the ear with direct activation of the vagus nerve produces an anti-anxiety effect that is important in the treatment of such conditions.

Wen (26) reported with electro-acupuncture an induced sense of well-being and suppression of the symptoms of sympathetic hyperactivity seen upon withdrawal of opiates. Ng (115, 116), of the National Institute of Health also reported that such ear electro-stimulation reduced the withdrawal symptoms of addiction. Such work has led to the wide use of ear acupuncture for help with other addictive behavior with such substances as alcohol, nicotine (smoking) and food (obesity).

Acupuncture is not a replacement for surgical anesthesia. At best it will play a very small role in Western surgery, despite the fact that it has much to recommend it. Acupuncture produces analgesia but not true anesthesia. Thus, the patient is aware of sensations other than pain and in some cases the pain itself is not entirely abolished but is only reduced in intensity. While this may be of great benefit to some patients, allowing them to avoid the common complications and discomfort that occur with general anesthesia, there are risks and inconveniences that Western surgeons are loath to assume. Relaxation is poor, especially when abdominal incisions are required. Anxious patients become even more so when placed in the strangeness of a surgical amphitheater. The procedure is more time consuming than usual anesthesia and is limited to those who are good acupuncture responders. A general anesthetic may be needed at some time during some operations.

Table VI lists the conditions suggested by the World Health Organization as amenable to acupuncture treatment. The list was given without statistics or proof of effectiveness and is thus simply a statement of common practice in some parts of the world. There have been many reports of single or multiple cases of all of these types of illness treated with some success. These reports appear scattered throughout the literature, many in the books of traditional acupuncture and in acupuncture journals such as the *American Journal of Chinese Medicine* and *American Journal of Acupuncture.* Many such reports are couched in metaphysical language, refer to traditional acupuncture theory and have no semblance of acceptable scientific standards for publication. Others do give a comparison of results with standard medical treatment practices. The percentage of success seems to depend upon whether the cases treated are acute or chronic. Most of our patients have been seen after contemporary medical treatments have failed. With this chronic population we have reported a 50% relief of pain in approximately half of the patients treated (33).

Series of cases reported in the literature stating significant improvement in up to 90% of patients treated, probably include numerous acutely ill patients who came to acupuncture as an initial mode of treatment for illnesses that were essentially self-limited. One of the most widely circulated tabulations of the success of acupuncture treatments is found in the writings of Felix Mann (98). He compiled the treatment results of 10 doctors who reported on 1,000 patients. Forty-four percent of patients were listed as "cured or markedly improved" and 20% showed moderate improvement for a total of 64% of patients who benefited from acupuncture treatments. Mann also quotes the work of Bischko (121), including some 2, 812 patients of whom 36% had "good results" and 25% who were listed as "+ –" for a total of 61% of patients who were helped to some extent.

A larger more recent series was reported from the Washington, D.C. Acupuncture Center (122). Eighty percent of patients were listed as having significant improvement out of 11,982 treated, while an additional 15% had slight improvement. The author states that the methods for collection of this information were "not entirely objective and scientific."

TABLE VI

MEDICAL CONDITIONS FOR WHICH ACUPUNCTURE IS COMMONLY USED

BRONCHITIS AND ASTHMA	CONJUNCTIVITIS
CORONARY HEART DISEASE	ACUTE AND CHRONIC RHINITIS
HYPERTENSION	ACUTE TONSILITIS
PEPTIC ULCER	ARTHRITIS
DISEASE OF THE BILIARY TRACT	SHOULDER PAIN
GASTROENTERITIS (ACUTE AND CHRONIC)	STRAINED NECK
DYSMENORRHEA	TENOSYNOVITIS
IRREGULAR MENSTRUATION	HEADACHE
MORNING SICKNESS	LUMBAGO (ACUTE AND CHRONIC)
ACUTE SIMPLE APPENDICITIS	SCIATICA
URTICARIA	TRIGEMINAL NEURALGIA
INTERCOSTAL NEURALGIA AND HERPES ZOSTER	FACIAL NERVE PARALYSIS
NEURASTHENIA	TOOTHACHE
ENURESIS	ACUTE SPRAINS OF SOFT TISSUES
VERTIGO	SEQUELAE OF CEREBROVASCULAR ACCIDENTS

From: Bannerman, R.H.: *The World Health Organization's Viewpoint on Acupuncture.* *Amer. J. Acupuncture*, 1980, 8:231-236.

The National Institute of Health's special ad hoc committee met to consider the many suggested uses of acupuncture. As reported by Howard Jenerick (123), "clinical investigators at eight separate pain clinics reported on acupuncture versus placebo treatments of acute and chronic pain in over 400 patients. Individual complaints and diagnoses ranged over a wide spectrum including phantom limb pain, causalgia and other neuropathy, headache and migraine, rheumatoid and osteo-arthritic pain, musculo-skeletal pain, etc. In many of these instances, the patients had experienced failure with conventional treatments and had been referred to the pain clinic by their original attending physician. On the order of 60% of all patients reported good to excellent relief from their pain for periods ranging from hours to months. Results varied according to the underlying pathology. The best outcome was obtained with self-limiting diseases, although some conditions of long standing (i.e., chronic headache, arthritis, low back pain) also responded well."

Matsumoto, Professor of Surgery and Director of Surgical Research at Hahnemann Medical College, Philadelphia, conducted single and double blind studies of the efficacy of acupuncture in the treatment of chronic neck and shoulder pain due to osteo-arthritis (12). He concluded that acupuncture was effective and that there was a statistically significant difference between the patients who received acupuncture at specific points and those who were stimulated at non-specific points.

Mendelson (90) reviewed published reports on the use of acupuncture in the treatment of chronic pain. He looked at both controlled and uncontrolled studies. Among 765 patients in six uncontrolled clinical reports there was a 70% improvement reported. In six controlled studies involving 417 patients, the reports showed equal success with placebo and acupuncture in four studies and a significantly higher percentage of patients improved by the use of acupuncture over and above placebo in two of the studies. Mendelson felt that there are few studies of acupuncture that meet high standards for validity. Nonetheless he stated that: "...on balance of evidence it appears that acupuncture has a place in the management of chronic pain resistant to orthodox treatment measures."

Mendelson's conclusion, which agrees essentially with our own belief, states: "...results of studies on the effect of acupuncture on pain threshold in man, and the use of acupuncture analgesia for surgical procedures all tend to support the conclusion that acupuncture has a marked analgesic effect: although most writers on this subject tend to stress either the "physical" or the "psychological" as being responsible for the analgesic effect, it is becoming apparent that a comprehensive theory of acupuncture analgesia will have to consider both physiological and psychological mechanisms."

In summary, it would appear that acupuncture is best used for the treatment of all types of pain both acute and chronic. For such conditions the clinical results will often be very good. Usually both physiological and psychological factors will be at work. Acupuncture is the treatment of choice for pain conditions. Here it has a chance of producing some lasting relief as compared to the short term effect of pain suppressing analgesics. These latter invariably show a propensity for side effects and addiction which are not present with acupuncture.

For other, non-pain, conditions acupuncture should be reserved for use in those illnesses that have not responded favorably to usual Western type treatment methods. It is essential that the decision to treat patients by acupuncture be made by medically trained persons who are in a position to determine whether the condition is indeed suitable for a treatment such as acupuncture or whether some other type of treatment might be more appropriate. This is especially true in serious illnesses where some more conventional type of treatment needs to be rapidly instituted to save life or to prevent additional suffering that might develop with the delay occasioned were reliance placed solely upon acupuncture. Often acupuncture can be effectively used in combination with some other types of treatment for the best results. In the final analysis acupuncture is but one of many medical treatments from among which the physician may select. When used properly it can significantly add to the therapeutic armamentarium.

VIII

ACUPUNCTURE AND WESTERN MEDICINE — LEGAL ASPECTS

In many parts of the world it is accepted that acupuncture is effective for pain relief and some other conditions. Sufficient medical experimental evidence exists to replace fanciful yin/yang explanations, developed in prescientific times, by facts and theories concordant with known mechanisms of nerve conduction and synaptic neurochemistry. Why then has Western medicine been reluctant to embrace acupuncture as a useful addition to the therapeutic armamentarium?

First of all, acupuncture was thrust into Western prominence in an unfavorable manner. Most medical innovations come from laboratory experiments and are given some prolonged preliminary testing and evaluation, both at the animal and clinical level. They are then announced to the public press, via scientists, physicians and medical schools. Acupuncture had no such introduction. It had its origin in folk medicine, shrouded in centuries of oriental mysticism, numerology and metaphysics. It was brought to public attention in the United States by the news media with great fanfare. It caught the public fancy and was widely taunted as a medical miracle and cure-all before the medical profession was aware of the full implications as a method of treatment. A demand for acupuncture rapidly developed throughout the Western world yet there was no place that physicians could readily acquire scientific training in this treatment technique. Available books were simply translations of centuries old mystical beliefs of alterations in some mysterious energy flow through the body. Such a belief in mysterious body energies is part and parcel of the ritual in many ancient healing practices. To scientifically trained M.D.'s this appeared as so much mumbo jumbo.

Shortly, after its reintroduction into the United States, there began to appear from the People's Republic of China reports of experimental work strongly indicating mechanisms within the central nervous system which offered scientifically acceptable theories of acupuncture's action. These theories were as conclusive as the theoretical bases of many treatments used in medical practice today. Such scientific evidence could well have justified the inclusion of acupuncture within the physicians' armamentarium but only a few physicians ventured into this field and the official stand of American medicine remained a negative one.

With lifting of the "bamboo curtain," some physicians toured China to see for themselves acupuncture in its traditional setting. Many were unable to explain what they saw, labeled acupuncture a Chinese form of hypnotic induction and summarily dismissed it as a treatment method. Opportunists and fringe medical groups soon sensed the growing demand for acupuncture. Unhampered by the necessity for explanations based on scientific reality, they accepted the metaphysical explanations of acupuncture and quickly opened shop. These occurrences further served to alienate physicians.

Skepticism concerning a new (or recently re-introduced) treatment is characteristic of the medical profession while just the opposite appears to be the case with non-scientifically trained laymen and health practitioners. In all peoples throughout the world there has always been a strong belief in mysticism and the occult. Such belief is strengthened by the hope and desire to find some miracle remedy to relieve pain and chronic suffering, especially when these symptoms have not responded well to traditional medical treatments.

It was probably the spectre of quackery that moved the AMA to expel acupuncture from their grace of approval and as recently as July, 1981, the House of Delegates of the American Medical Association took a stand, calling acupuncture an "unproven modality of therapy."* This stance is unfortunate as it has discouraged many physicians from taking a closer look at acupuncture — an action that might have led them to an awareness of some of the scientific investigations that are underway and to have considered trying it in their own practices. Thus the AMA's "official" stand which was taken to protect the public from unproven therapies may actually have served to further promote the use of acupuncture by persons without proper medical training.

This danger was pointed out at the November, 1975 annual meeting of The Federation of State Medical Boards (35). At that time, I stated that "to establish boards to examine candidates in the ancient philosophical concepts of Chinese medicine in this age of scientific enlightenment is, indeed, but a travesty".

As of January, 1980 (36), six states, California, Hawaii, Montana, Nevada, New York and Rhode Island, issued licenses to non-medical persons for the unsupervised practice of acupuncture. The requirements for certification varies from 50 to 500 hours of teaching or the possession of credentials established by boards stressing the metaphysics of oriental medicine. Six other states, Maryland, Massachusetts, Oregon, South Carolina, Tennessee and Washington issue licenses to non-medical per-

---

**American Medical News*, July, 1981

sons to practice acupuncture under medical supervision. Forty-three states have ruled that acupuncture is the practice of medicine or dentistry. Fourteen of these require that M.D.'s and D.O.'s must have special training in traditional Chinese medicine. These are: Alabama, Connecticut, Delaware, Florida, Georgia, Illinois, Louisiana, Maryland, New York, Ohio, Oklahoma, Utah, Virginia and Washington. Four that require special training for M.D.'s and D.O.'s also license non-medical acupuncturists (Maryland, New York, Oregon and Washington). In the remaining states M.D.'s and D.O.'s can practice acupuncture without special training or licensure. As the pressure for licensure by non-medical persons is continuing and strong, the legal status in several states is in flux at the time of this writing.

It is our opinion that, for reasons of patient safety, acupuncture should be under medical supervision and it is hoped that the facts revealed in this book will demonstrate that safe and useful acupuncture can be practiced by any physician with the basic knowledge of anatomy and physiology learned in medical school.

The crucial question to be asked of state licensing boards is: "who is qualified to diagnose and design the treatment plan for recognizable symptoms and disease?" The only acceptable answer, in the light of modern medical knowledge, is a person trained and licensed to practice the healing arts. If acupuncture is properly defined as one of those healing arts then acupuncture should be placed under medical supervision. The word acupuncture means puncture of the body by means of a sharp instrument. This is a common medical procedure. If the proper placement of acupuncture needles depends upon neurophysiological concepts such as are taught in every medical school, then it is no more consistent to demand special certification for this procedure than it is to require special certification for a physician to do venapuncture or lumbar puncture. These latter procedures are permissible under any blanket license to practice medicine or osteopathy.

Until some change is made in the laws of those few states where special examination and certification is required for the practice of "acupuncture", physicians who do not wish to go through an outlandish examination in the theory of ancient Chinese medicine might well be advised to announce that they practice "modern physiologic acupuncture" as opposed to "ancient traditional Chinese acupuncture." Warren has suggested the term "dermal puncture" (37), and we have often referred to our work as "percutaneous electrical nerve stimulation".

A recent article from the Hasting's Report (38), points to an even greater danger to good patient care that has evolved from the confusion over certification of acupuncturists. Being zealous to protect the fundamental right of privacy, a Federal Court Judge in Texas ruled that the application of the Texas Medical Practice Act to limit the practice of acupuncture to duly licensed physicians was an unconstitutional invasion of an individual's right to seek the treatment of his/her choice. This Texas statute, that was so weakened, is typical of existing statutes in the 50 states that have permitted state medical licensing boards the salutory effect of outlawing the sale of quack cancer cures and the practice of other types of charlatinism. As of now the court's opinion stands unchallenged and thus it may well act to subsequently weaken the traditional role of medicine to protect the health and safety of all citizens. The author of this article quoted my own recent report in the JAMA (39), as supporting the medical establishment's "regulatory scheme" in that I presented acupuncture as a scientific treatment method for use by physicians. This prompted my response in the form of a letter to the editor (40) in which I point out the abysmal lack of evidence that was before the court regarding a "scientific physiologic" form of acupuncture that differed from the "ancient traditional" approach. The court was apparently unaware of abuses that had already been reported from malpractice by inept acupuncturists such as infected needles that resulted in limb amputations, collapsed lungs from improper needle placement and misdiagnoses that cause untold harm and suffering. It is my hope that knowledge of a scientifically based acupuncture by properly trained medical personnel will lead to corrective judicial and legislative action.

There is another problem faced by the physician who plans to start using acupuncture. This is in regard to the FDA's regulations concerning the equipment to be used for acupuncture treatments. Electronic stimulators and needles used in acupuncture are labeled as "experimental devices". This may present a problem for physicians who wish to import treatment apparatus such as that available from sources within the People's Republic of China.

A final consideration is the question of malpractice coverage for physicians performing acupuncture as some carriers have not yet included it in their rate schedules. Also, acupuncture does not yet have a widely recognized scientific basis so other carriers may be hesitant to cover it or may require additional premiums. In this regard, I would quote the opinion of Dr. William Dornette, M.D., Director of Education and Research, Division of Anesthesiology at the Cleveland Clinic in Cleveland, Ohio (41). "Having observed and administered acupuncture, I sincerely believe that the use of this technique by a licensed practitioner who has had training in acupuncture and has a thorough knowledge in anatomy poses no more, and certainly far less, risk to the patient than many other therapeutic modalities." It is however to be recommended that all patients receiving acupuncture sign a release form indicating the novel nature of this form of treatment, spelling out possible, though rare, complications, alternate modes of treatment for the condition under consideration, and, as well, that in the U.S., acupuncture is often used on a research basis.

REFERENCES TO TEXT

1. Spiegel, H., and Spiegel, D.: *Trance and Treatment.* Basic Books, New York, 1978.
2. Kroger, W.S.: Hypnotism and Acupuncture. *JAMA*, 1972, 220:1012.
3. Wall, P.: An eye on the needle. *New Scientist*, 1972, 55:129-131.
4. Wall, P.: Acupuncture revisited. *New Scientist*, 1974, 64:31-34.
5. Katz, R.L., Kao, C.Y., Spiegel, H., and Katz, G.T.: Acupuncture and Hypnosis. *Advances in Neurology*, 1974, 4:819-825.
6. Katz, R.: In, Jenerick, H.P., *Proceedings of the National Institutes of Health Acupuncture Research Conf.* Bethesda, Md., 1973, p. 109.
7. Knox, J., Hanfield-Jones, C.D., and Shum, K.: Subject Expectancy and the Reduction of Cold Pressor Pain with Acupuncture and Placebo Acupuncture. *Psychosom. Med.*, 1979, 41:477-486.
8. Lu, Gwei-Djen and Needham, J.: *Celestial Lancets.* Cambridge University Press, 1980, p. 427.
9. Moore, M.E., and Berk, S.N.: Acupuncture for Chronic Shoulder Pain. *Ann.Int. Med.*, 1976, 84:381-384.
10. Kepes, E.R., Chen, M., and Schapira, M.: A Critical Evaluation of Acupuncture in the Treatment of Pain. *Adv. in Pain Res. Ther.*, 1976, 1:817-822.
11. Omura, Y.: Editorial. Historical Aspects of Acupuncture. *Acup. and Electro-Therapeutics Res.*, 1975-76, I(1-4), p. 17.
12. Matsumoto, T.: *Acupuncture for Physicians.* C.C. Thomas, Springfield, Ill., 1974, pp. 204.
13. Collison, D.: Acupuncture and Hypnotherapy. *Med. J. Australia*, 1974, 2(3):112.
14. Nemerof, H., and Rothman, I.: Acupuncture and Hypnotism. *Amer. J. Clin. Hypn.*, 1974, 16(3):156-159.
15. Frost, E.A.: Acupuncture and Hypnosis. Apples and Oranges. *New York State J. Med.*, 1978, 78(11):1768-72.
16. MacHovec, F.J., and Man, S.C.: Acupuncture and Hypnosis Compared in 58 cases. *Amer. J. Clin. Hypn.*, 1978, 21(1):45-47.
17. Andersson, S.A., and Holmgren, E.: On Acupuncture Analgesia and the Mechanism of Pain. *Amer. J. Chinese Med.*, 1975, 3:311.
18. Goldstein, A., and Hilgard, E.R.: Failure of the Opiate Antagonist Nalaxone to Modify Hypnotic Analgesia. *Proc. Nat. Acad. Sci.*, 1975, 72:2041.
19. Wen, H.C., and Teo, S.W.: Experience in the Treatment of Drug Addiction by Electro-Acupuncture. *Mod. Med. Asia*, 1975, 11:23-24.
20. Patterson, M. (as quoted in Potterton, D.A.): Ten Day Cure for Addition. *Bestways*, 1981, 9(3):104-105.
21. Han, C.S., Tang, J., Jen, M.F., Zhou, A.F., Fan, S.G., and Qio, X.C.: The Role of Central Neurotransmitters in Acupuncture Analgesia. Private Publication, *Research Group of Acupuncture Anesthesia.* Peking, P.R.C.
22. Gunn, C.C.: *Pain, Acupuncture and Related Subjects.* From: Workers' Compensation Board of British Columbia. Privately published, 828 West Broadway, Vancouver, B.C. V521J8.
23. Melzack, R., and Wall, P.: Pain Mechanism: A New Theory. *Science*, 1965, 150:971-73.
24. Brown, M.L., Ulett, G.A., and Stern, J.A.: Acupuncture Loci: Techniques for Location. *Amer. J. Chinese Med.*, 1974, 2(1):67-74.

25. Liu, Y.K., Varela, M., and Oswald, R.: The Correspondence Between Some Motor Points and Acupuncture Loci. *Amer. J. Chinese Med.*, 1975, 3:347-358.
26. Brown, M.L., Ulett, G.A., and Stern, J.A.: The Effects of Acupuncture on White Blood Cell Counts. *Amer. J. Chinese Med.*, 1974, 2(4):383-398.
27. Levine, J.D., Gordon, N.C., and Fields, H.L.: The Mechanism of Placebo Analgesia. *The Lancet*, 1978, 35:654-657.
28. Omura, Y.: Pathophysiology of Acupuncture Treatment: Effects of Acupuncture on Cardiovascular and Nervous Systems. *Acup. and Electro-Therapeutics Res.*, 1975, 1:51-140.
29. Saletu, B., Saletu, M., Brown, M., Stern, J.A., Sletten, I.W., and Ulett, G.A.: Hypno-Analgesia and Acupuncture Analgesia: A Neurophysiologic Reality: *Neuropsychobiology*, 1975, 1:218-242.
30. Parwatikar, S., Brown, M., Stern, J., Ulett, G.A., and Sletten, I.W.: Acupuncture, Hypnosis and Experimental Pain. I. Study with Volunteers. *Acup. and Electro-Therapeutics Res. J.*, 1978, 3:161-190.
31. Ulett, G., Parwatikar, S., Stern, J.A., and Brown, M.: Acupuncture, Hypnosis and Experimental Pain. II. Study with Patients. *Acup. and Electro-Therapeutics Res. J.* 1978, 3:191-201.
32. Ulett, G.A.: (Editorial). Acupuncture: Pricking the Bubble of Skepticism. *Biol. Psych.*, 1978, 13:159-161.
33. Ulett, G.A.: Control of Chronic Pain by Acupuncture. *Psych. J. Univ. of Ottawa*, 1977, 2(3):143-146.
34. Kerr, F.W.L.: The Structural Basis of Pain. Circuitry and Pathways. In, Ng, L., Lorenz, K.Y. and Bonica, J.J.: *Pain, Discomfort and Humanitarian Care.* Elsevier, North Holland, 1980, pp. 49-60.
35. Ulett, G.A.: Acupuncture, A Technique for the Regularly Licensed Physician. *Federation Bulletin*, Federation of State Medical Boards of the U.S. 1975, 62(11), 334-343.
36. Acquah, J.S.: *The Legal Status of Acupuncture in the United States.* Synthesis Production, P.O. Box 842, Newhall, Ca. 91321.
37. Warren, F.Z.: *Handbook of Medical Acupuncture.* Van Nostrand Reinhold Co., New York, 1976, pp. 273.
38. Schwartz, R.: *Yin, Yang and the Right to Privacy. Acupuncture and Expertise. A Challenge to Physician Control.* The Hastings Center Report, April, 1981, p. 5-7.
39. Ulett, G.: Acupuncture Treatment for Pain Relief. *JAMA*, 1981, 245:768-769.
40. Ulett, G.: *Quack-u-puncture or Cure?* The Hastings Center Reports, 1982, 12:45.
41. Dornette, W.H.L.: Acupuncture and the Law. In, Warren, F.Z., *Handbook of Medical Acupuncture*, Van Nostrand Reinhold Co., New York, 1976.
42. Chang, H.T.: Integrative Action of Thalamus in the Process of Acupuncture for Analgesia. *Scientia Sinica*, 1973, 16:25-60.
43. Melzack, R., Melinkoff, R.F.: Analgesia Produced by Brain Stimulation. Evidence of a Prolonged Onset Period. *Exp. Neurol., 1974, 43:369-374.*
44. Yao, T., Andersson, S., and Thoren, P.: *Long Lasting Cardiovascular Depression Induced by Acupuncture-Like Stimulation of the Sciatic Nerve in Unanesthetized Spontaneously Hypersensitive Rats.* 1981, in press.
45. Andersson, S., Shyu, B., and Thoren, P.: *Physiological Significance of Acupuncture Stimulation.* 1981, in press.
46. Kostrubala, T.: *The Joy of Running.* New York, J.B. Lippincott, 1976, p. 129.

47. Pomeranz, B., Cheng, R., Law, P.: Acupuncture Reduces Electrophysiological and Behavioral Responses to Noxious Stimuli Pituitary is Implicated. *Exp. Neurol.*, 1977, 54:172-178.
48. Roos, A., Rydenhag, G., and Andersson, S.A.: Activity in Cortical Cells After Stimulation of Tooth Pulp Afferents in the Cat. Extracellular Analysis. *Pain*, 1981, submitted for publication.
49. Roos, A., Rydenberg, B., and Andersson, S.A.: Cortical Responses Evoked by Tooth Pulp Stimulation in the Cat. Surface and Intracortical Responses. *Pain*, 1981, submitted for publication.
50. Andersson, S.A., Roos, A., and Rydenhag, B.: Activity in Cortical Cells After Stimulation of Tooth Pulp Afferents in the Cat. Intracellular Analysis. *Pain*, 1981, submitted for publication.
51. Roos, A., and Rydenhag, B.: Effects of Low Frequency Conditioning Stimulation on Cortical Potentials Evoked by Noxious Stimulation. *Pain*, 1981, submitted for publication.
52. Peking Acupuncture Anesthesia Coordinating Group. Preliminary Study on the Mechanism of Acupuncture Anesthesia. *Scientia Sinica*, 1973, 16:447-456.
53. Chatrian, G.E., Camfield, R.C., and Knauss, T.A.: Cerebral Responses to Electrical Tooth Pulp Stimulation in Man. An Objective Correlate of Acute Experimental Pain. *Neurology*, 1975, 25:745-757.
54. Lassen, N.A., Ingvar, D.H., and Skinh, J.E.: Brain Function and Blood Flow. *Sci. Am.*, 1978, Oct., 50-59.
55. Mayer, D.J.: The Centrifugal Control of Pain. In, Ng, L., and Bonica, JJ. *Pain, Discontent and Humanitarian Care.* Elsevier, North Holland, 1980, 83-105.
56. Pert, C., and Snyder, S.: Opiate Receptor: Demonstration in Nervous Tissue. *Science*, 1973, 179:1011-1014.
57. Simon, E.J., Heller, J.M., Edelman, I.: Stereospecific Binding of the Potent Narcotic Analgesic (3H) Etorphine to Rat Brain Homogenete. *Proc. Nat. Acad. Sci.*, 1973, 70:1947.
58. Terenius, L.: Characteristics of the "Receptor" for Narcotic Analgesics in Synpatic Plasma Membrane Fraction from Rat Brain, ACTA. *Pharmacol. Toxicol.*, 1973, 33:377-384.
59. Hughes, J.: Isolation of an Endogenous Compound from the Brain with Pharmacological Properties Similar to Morphine. *Brain Res.*, 1975, 88:295-308.
60. Mayer, J.D., Prig, D.D., and Raffi, A.: Antagonism of Acupuncture Analgesia in Man by the Narcotic Antagonist Naloxone. *Brain Res.*, 1977, 14:368-372.
61. Barber, J., and Mayer, D.J.: Evaluation of the Efficacy and Neural Mechanism of a Hypnotic Analgesia Procedure in Experimental and Clinical Dental Pain. *Pain*, 1977, 4:41-48.
62. Goldstein, A., and Hilgard, E.R.: Failure of the Opiate Antagonist Naloxone to Modify Hypnotic Analgesia. *Proc. Nat. Acad. Sci.*, 1975, 72:2041-2043.
63. Singry, B., and Benassi, V.A.: Occult Beliefs. *Amer. Sci.*, 1981, 69:49-55.
64. Chiang, Chen-Yu, Chiang, Chhing-Tshai, et al.: Peripheral Afferent Pathways for Acupuncture Analgesia. *SCISA*, 1973 (16 Nov.) 210.
65. Evans, R.: Smythe Clinic. Personal Communication. Reported by Needham, J., and Lu, Gwei-Djen: *Celestial Lancets*, Cambridge University Press, 1980, p. 249.
66. Stewart, D., Thompson, J., and Oswald, I.: Acupuncture Analgesia: An Experimental Investigation. *Brit. Med. J.*, 1977, 67, ptl. (#6053).

67. Noordenbos, W.: *Pain*. Elsevier, Amsterdam, 1959.
68. Wall, P.D.: The Gate Control Theory of Pain Mechanisms. A Re-examination, and Re-statement. *Brain*, 1978, 101-1-18.
69. Chang Hsiang-Thung: Integrative Action of the Thalamus in the Process of Acupuncture Analgesia. *SCISA*, 1973, 16 (No.), *AJCM*, 1974 2 (no 1) 1.
70. Gracely, R.H.: Pain Measurement in Man. In, Ng, L., and Bonica, J.J.: *Pain, Discomfort and Humanitarian Care*. Elsevier/North Holland, 1981, pp. 111-137.
71. Loeser, J.D.: Nonpharmacological Approaches to Pain Relief. In, Ng, L., and Bonica, J.J.: *Pain Discomfort and Humanitarian Care*. Elsevier/North Holland, 1981, 275-292.
72. Sweet, W.H.: Some current problems in pain research and therapy (including Needle Puncture), "Acupuncture", Part II Second J.J. Bonica Lecture. *Pain*, 1981, 10:297-309.
73. Zhang, A.Z., Pan, X.P., Xu, S.F., Cheng, J.S., and Mo, W.Y.: Endorphins and Acupuncture Analgesia. *J. Chinese Med.*, 1980, 93:673-680.
74. Sjolund, B., Terenius, L., and Erikson, M.: Increased Cerebrospinal Fluid Levels of Endorphins After Electro-Acupuncture. *Acta Physiol. Scand.*, 1977, 100:382-384.
75. Wancura, I., and Konig, G.: On the Neurophysiological Explanation of Acupuncture Analgesia. *Amer. J. Chinese Med.*, 1974, 2:193-198.
76. Ha, H., and Tan, E.C.: Sensory Representation of Acupuncture Site in the Cortex of the Monkey. *Anatomical Record*, 1981, 99(3):103-A.
77. Nakatani, Y.: A Guide for the Application of Ryodoraku Autonomous Nerve Regulatory Therapy. 1972, Tokyo, Japan.
78. Gaito, J.: The Kindling Effect. *Physiological Psychology*, 1965, 2:45-50.
79. Lorente de No, R.: Analysis of the activity of Chains of Internuncial Neurons. *J. Neurophysiol.*, 1938, 1:207-244.
80. Dusser de Barenne, J.G., and McCulloch, W.S.: Factors for Facilitation and Extinction in the Central Nervous System. *J. Neurophysiol.*, 1939, 2:319-355.
81. Loeser, J.D., Ward, A.A., and White, L.E.: Chronic Deafferentation of Human Spinal Cord Neurons. *J. Neurosurg.*, 1968, 29:48-50.
82. Livingston, W.K.: *Pain Mechanisms*. The MacMillan Co., New York, 1943, pp. 253.
83. Omura, Y.: Patho-Physiology of Acupuncture Treatment: Effects of Acupuncture on Cardiovascular and Nervous Systems. *Acupuncture and Electro-Therap. Res. J.*, 1975, 1:51-140.
84. Yao, T., Andersson, S., and Thoren, P.: Influence of a Prolonged Low Frequency Electrical Stimulation of Somatic Afferents on Autonomic Functions and Pain Threshold in Unanesthetized Rats. In Press.
85. MacKenzie, J.: *Symptoms and Their Interpretations*. Shaw and Sons, London, 1912, 304.
86. Kellgren, J.H.: On the Distribution of Pain Arising from Deep Somatic Structures with Charts of Segmental Pain Areas. *Clin. Sci.*, 1939-42, 4:35-46.
87. Head, H.: On Disturbances of Sensation with Especial Reference to the Pain of Visceral Diseases. *Brain*, 1893, 16:1-133.
88. Tam, K.C., and Yin, H.K.: The Effect of Acupuncture on Essential Hypertension. *Amer. J. Chinese Med.*, 1975, 3:369-375.
89. Liao, S.J.: Recent Advances in the Understanding of Acupuncture. *Yale J. Biol. and Med.*, 1978, 51:55-65.
90. Mendelson, G.: Acupuncture and Cholinergic Suppression of Withdrawal Symptoms: An Hypothesis. *Brit. J. Addiction*, 1978, 75:166-170.
91. Britt, A.A.: *The Basic Writings of Sigmund Freud*. Random House, 1938, 1001.
92. Olds, J.: Self-stimulation of the Brain. *Science*, 1958, 127:315-324.

93. Weitzman, E., Boyar, R.M., Kapen, S., and Hellman, L.: The Relationship of Sleep and Sleep Stages to Neuroendocrine Secretion and Biological Rhythms in Man. *Recent Progress in Hormone Research*, 1975, 31:399-446.
94. Hartman, E.: Tryptophan in Psychiatry and Neurology. A Symposium Presented at the III World Congress of Biological Psychiatry, Stockholm, Sweden, June 28-July 3, 1981.
95. Brown, M.L., Ulett, G.A., and Stern, J.A.: Acupuncture Loci: Techniques for Location. *Amer. J. Chinese Med.*, 1974, 2(1):67-74.
96. Liu, Y.H., Varela, M., Oswald, R.: The Correspondence Between Some Motor Points and Acupuncture Loci. *Amer. J. Chinese Med.*, 1975, 3:347-358.
97. Liao, S.J.: Acupuncture Points, Concordance with Motor Points of Skeletal Muscles. *Arch. Phys. Med. Rehab.*, 1975, 56:550.
98. Mann, F.: *Scientific Aspects of Acupuncture*. William Heinemann Medical Books, Ltd., London, 1977, 77.
99. Mendelson, G.: Acupuncture Analgesia. II. Review of Current Theories. *Aust., N.Z. J. Med.*, 1978, 8:100-105.
100. Anon: The Relation Between Acupuncture Analgesia and Neurotransmitters in Rabbit Brain. *China Med. J.*, 1973, 8:105.
101. Reiderer, P., Tenk, H., Werner, H., Bischko, J., Rett, A., and Krisper, H.: Manipulation of Neurotransmitters by Acupuncture. *J. Neural Transmission*, 1975, 37:81.
102. Chang, C.Y., Chang, C.T., et al: Peripheral Efferent Pathways for Acupuncture Analgesia. *Scientia Sineca*, 1973, 16:210-217.
103. Chang Hsiang-Tung: People's Republic of China Acupuncture Anesthesia. Colored Movies. 1973.
104. Weiss, S., and Davis, D.: Significance of Afferent Impulses from Skin in Mechanism of Visceral Pain: Skin Infiltration as Useful Therapeutic Measure. *Amer. J. M. Sci.*, 1928, 176:517-536.
105. Acupuncture Anesthesia Research Group, Morphology Unit, Peking Medical College, Peking. Survey of Electric Resistance of Rabbitt's Pinna in Experimental Peritonitis and Peptic Ulcer. *Chinese Med. J.*, New Series: 1976, 2:423-434.
106. Travell, J., and Rinzler, S.H.: Relief of Cardiac Pain by Local Block of Somatic Trigger Areas. *Proc. Soc. Exptl. Biol. Med.*, 1946, 63:480-482.
107. Travell, J., and Rinzler, S.H.: The Myofascial Genesis of Pain. Scientific Exhibit shown at Annual Session of American Medical Association. Atlantic City, 1951. *Postgrad. Med.*, 1952, 2:425-434.
108. Travell, J.: Referred Pain from Skeletal Muscle. *New York State J. Med.*, 1955, 55:331-340.
109. Melzack, R., Stillwell, D.M., and Fox, I.J.: Trigger Points and Acupuncture Points for Pain: Correlation and Implications. *Pain*, 1977, 3:3-23.
110. Wu Wei-Ping: *Chinese Acupuncture*. Translation by Philip M. Chancellor, Health Science Press, Rustington, Sussex, England, 1959, 181.
111. Gunn, C.C., and Millbrandt, W.E.: The Neurological Mechanism of Needle-Grasp in Acupuncture. *Amer. J. Acup.*, 1977, 5:115-120.
112. Bowsher, D.: Role of the Reticular Formation in Responses to Noxious Stimulation. *Pain*, 1976, 2:361-378.
113. Vierck, C.J., Jr., Lineberry, C.G., Lee, P.K., et al: Prolonged hyperalgesia Following Acupuncture in Monkeys. *Life Science*, 1974, 15:1277-1289.
114. Ulett, G.: Acupuncture is not Hypnosis — Physiological Studies. *Amer. J. Acupuncture*, 1982, in press.

115. Ng, L.K.Y., Douthitt, T.C., Thoa, N.B., et al: Modification of morphine withdrawal syndrome in rats following transauricular electrostimulation: an experimental paradigm for auricular electroacupuncture. *Biol. Psychiat.*, 1975, 10:575-580.
116. Ng, L.K.Y: Acupuncture in the Management of Narcotic Dependency. A Presentation of Acupuncture. Conference Sponsored by the Ad Hoc Committee to Study Acupuncture. Connecticut State Medical Society, Farmington, Conn., September 29, 1975.
117. Shaar, C.J., Frederickson, R.C.A., and Dininger, N.B., et al: Enkephalin Analogues and Naloxone Modulate the Release of Growth Hormone and Prolactin — Evidence for Regulation by an Endogenous Opioid Peptide in Brain. *Life Science*, 1977, 21:853-850.
118. Cocchi, D., Santagostino, A., Gil-Ad, I., et al: Leu-enkephalin-stimulated growth hormone with Prolactin Release in the Rat: Comparison with the Effect of Morphine. *Life Science*, 1977, 20:2041 2045.
119. Dupont, A., Cusan, L., Garon, M., et al: Beta-endorphin Stimulation of Growth Hormone Release in vivo. *Proc. Natl. Acad. Sci.*, USA, 1977, 74-358-359.
120. River, C., Vale, W., Ling, N., et al: Stimulation in vivo of the Secretion of Prolactin and Growth Hormone by B-Endorphin. *Endocrinol.*, 1977, 100:238-241.
121. Bischko, J.: From the Vienna Allgemaine Poliklinik as Reported by Felix Mann. In, *Acupuncture, the Ancient Chinese Art of Healing and How it Works Scientifically.* Vintage Books, 1973.
122. Wensel, L.O.: *Acupuncture in Medical Practice.* Reston Publishing Co., 1980, p. 333.
123. Jenerick, H.P.: The NIH Acupuncture Research Study. As reported in Warren, F.Z.: *Handbook of Medical Acupuncture.* Van Nostrand Reinhold Company, 1976, p. 273.

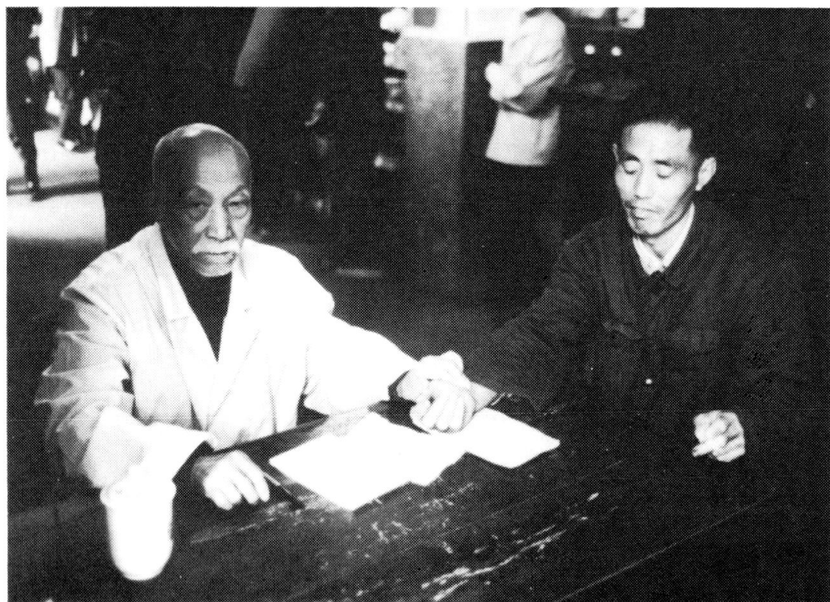

Figure 39. Traditional pulse diagnosis in an herb store in Wuhan, Peoples Republic of China, November 1980.

APPENDIX
TRADITIONAL CHINESE ACUPUNCTURE

SPREAD OF ACUPUNCTURE THROUGHOUT THE WORLD

The ancient technique of acupuncture dates back some 4,000 years. Its use has spread throughout the world such that today acupuncture holds an important position in the treatment of one third of the world's population.

From its origin in China, acupuncture spread to Korea by approximately 300 A.D. and then on to Japan by the 17th century. As trade with the Far East developed, European visitors came in contact with Chinese and Japanese physicians. In this manner, acupuncture was brought to the attention of Europeans at a time when Western medicine was concerned with the harsher practices of blistering, phlebotomy, purging and cautery. Some Western physicians of that time ridiculed the symbolic correlations of Chinese medical therapy with Eastern philosophy. Western medicine at that time was, however, equally empirically based and concerned with theories of demoniacal possession, the four body humors, astrology and other medieval vagueries.

By the year 1800, there was in Europe considerable interest in acupuncture. Berloiz, father of the composer, wrote the first French book on acupuncture in 1816, describing the treatment of many illnesses by this method. He particularly stressed the dramatic effects in the relief of muscle and joint pain. In 1825, Chevalier Sarlandiere first described the application of an electric current from Leyden jars applied to the inserted needles. It is reported that Gennai Hiraga of Envo, Japan, similarly used electro-acupuncture in 1764. In the early 1800's reports on the use of acupuncture came from both Germany and England. During the 1840's, Leed's Infirmary became a great center for the use of acupuncture in the treatment of rheumatism. From Europe interest in acupuncture spread to the United States as evidence is reported of its use as early as 1825. Mention was made of acupuncture in a surgical treatise by Billroth in 1863. In his, "Principles and Practice of Medicine," Sir William Osler, in 1912, recommended acupuncture for the treatment of sciatica.

While the use of acupuncture in Europe increased early in the 20th century, such was not the case in America. Reference to acupuncture was deleted from later editions of Osler's text and there was little known about it in America until the visit of President Nixon to China in 1972. It is noteworthy that while contemporary U.S. medicine had practically no knowledge of acupuncture, such services had been available for many years in the clinics and hospitals in France and England. Nogier of Lyon France was busy with his studies of ear acupuncture (auriculotherapy) in the 1950's and in 1962 Felix Mann of London published his widely read books on acupuncture. With the visit of President Nixon to China, Reston, a member of the press corps, required an appendectomy. An account of his relief from post-operative discomfort accomplished by acupuncture was widely publicized in the U.S. The idea that treatment by tiny needles could relieve pain quickly caught the public's fancy. With lifting of the bamboo curtain an increasing interest in things Oriental carried acupuncture to the forefront of newsworthy items. Medical teams visited China and returned with tales, not only of treatment of many illnesses and of relief from pain by acupuncture, but also of surgery done under acupuncture analgesia without the use of the usual gas anesthetics. Explanation of such phenomena in terms of yin/yang theory is unacceptable to U.S. physicians. They were quick to explain acupuncture in terms of hypnosis and Oriental stoicism and very few gave it serious consideration.

At this time in the U.S. there was a growing interest in holistic medicine — the prevention of illness and the treatment of disease without the use of drugs. Acupuncture fitted very nicely into this concept. The public's hope for miracle cures had been stirred by the press. Acupuncturists without medical training who were not disturbed by metaphysical explanations for medical treatments quickly moved in to meet the demand for acupuncture treatments. Without the legal and ethical constraints customary within organized medicine, exaggerated claims, pretentious advertising, acupuncture mills and other malpractice flourished.

Paradoxically, in laboratories throughout the world there was, at this time, an increased interest in pain research which included studies of the physiology and the biochemistry of acupuncture, electro-stimulation and endorphins. Sufficient evidence was accumulating to replace the traditional metaphysical theories with scientific explanations for the action of acupuncture. Some physicians became interested in applying these techniques for pain management. Such physician interest was minimal, however, and pressure from non-M.D.'s forced through legislation in several states whereby licensure to practice acupuncture depends upon training and examination in the ancient non-factual metaphysical theories. At the time of this writing training in acupuncture based upon modern techniques and physiological principles is essentially unavailable to practicing physicians and acupuncture is not yet a part of the curriculum of U.S. medical schools.

THEORETICAL CONCEPTS OF TRADITIONAL ACUPUNCTURE

There is an old Chinese proverb which states, "One generation opens the road upon which another generation travels". It is a tribute to those ancient Chinese physicians that some of the acupuncture points that they selected by trial and error coincide with now known anatomical structures. Many of their clinical observations have direct pertinence to current scientific concepts, though due to the almost non-existent scientific knowledge of that time they were couched in fanciful, metaphysical and numerological terms.

We have shown that it is possible to select points for needle insertion and stimulation on a rational, scientific basis and in accord with contemporary anatomical and neurophysiological knowledge and theory. The information that has made it possible to develop rational acupuncture techniques has become available from research laboratories mostly within the past two decades. Thus the great majority of persons doing acupuncture still have their practice and thinking based upon outmoded concepts. The books and journals available on the subject use theories and terminology derived from the historic Nei-Ching, a centuries-old medical manuscript (1).

In order to comprehend these writings and to communicate with other acupuncturists, a knowledge of some of these basic concepts of traditional Chinese medicine is necessary. As Chairman Mao believed, ancient Chinese medicine is truly a veritable storehouse from which may develop much that is useful to modern medicine.

Traditional acupuncture is based upon concepts of "energetic medicine" (2), a belief that there is a continous generation and flow of energy (chhi, life force) throughout the body. This force has two polarities, yin and yang. When the flow of these energies is thought to be in balance a condition of health exists. Illness occurs when they are out of balance. These energies travel through the body over 12 major channels (meridians), each linked to a particular organ or body function. On each meridian there exist numerous acupuncture points at which the flow of energy can be influenced by the insertion and manipulation of needles. Such needling (pique) can either strengthen (tonify) deficient energy in a given organ/system or weaken (disperse) excess energy.

A traditional acupuncturist must determine through a palpation of the 12 radial pulses which meridian is deficient in energy. Such pulse diagnosis was felt to be the means for detecting illness before actual symptoms of disease occurred (3). Thus acupuncture was used to correct the ying/yang balance and prevent illness. When symptoms of disease were already present it was felt that the existing pain and symptoms caused such a disturbance of body equilibrium that pulse diagnosis was of little use and the treatment was then placed on an inferior basis requiring only the placement of needles according to a "set formula" of points. Each formula was specific for a different illness. Once the illness had been corrected a master of acupuncture could discern from the pulse which meridian imbalance had caused the illness and could then determine the proper placement of the needles to prevent further malfunction.

The theoretical basis for treatment by acupuncture was developed from a consideration of the interrelationship of five elements or essential forces, each of which was related to a pair of organs. One set of organs was "hollow" (fu: small intestine, gall bladder, stomach, colon, urinary bladder, and triple heater), the other "solid" (tsang: heart, liver, spleen, lungs, kidney and pericardium). An elaborate set of rules governed the selection of treatment points utilizing not only a formula relating these five elements (meridians/organs) in terms of dominance and submission but as well the relationship of the elements to other cosmic forces: nature, color, sounds, etc. Lists of acupuncture points to be used were formulated in terms of their relationship to various cosmic forces and the waxing and waning of yin and yang strength at various times of the day.

The complexity of the metaphysical theory is such that it is said a lifetime was required to master the total system of acupuncture and, indeed, some of it was reported to be held as closely guarded secrets by masters of acupuncture or passed on within families from father to son. Inherent in the whole complex approach lies the concept of "balancing energies" or of bringing forces into harmony. Hence, the same point is felt to be of use to either increase or decrease a given function, depending upon the state of energy balance in the body at that time and the manner of stimulation used.

Acupuncture is but one part of traditional Chinese medicine. The use of herbs and other types of physical manipulation such as diet are equally important. The theoretical basis of Chinese medicine was built around attempts to explain health, illness and man's relationship to the universe at a time prior to recorded history. There was then but the barest knowledge of anatomy, practically no idea of physiology and in China, as elsewhere in the world, concepts of life, health and illness were based upon philosophic ideas, superstition and religion. Thus acupuncture theory is but a reflection of the beliefs of that period.

In keeping with Taoistic philosophy man was thought to be a microcosmic reflection of the cosmos. The central, single world force, perfect whole or Tao was the yin/yang consisting of two elements, yin and yang. These two opposing complimentary forces each stood for one of paired elements. As shown in Table I, all manner of opposites could be classified as being either yin or yang in nature.

TABLE I

VARIOUS PAIRS OF OPPOSITES CLASSIFIED AS YIN OR YANG

Yin	Yang
Earth	Heaven
Shadow	Sunlight
Female	Male
Cold	Hot
Weak	Powerful
Night	Day
Left Side	Right Side
Sinking	Rising
Abdomen	Back
Metal	Wood
Water	Fire
Sour & pungent	Sweet & bitter
Even numbers	Odd numbers
Ying energy (Constructive)	Wei energy (Destructive)

Yin/yang is traditionally diagrammed as a circle containing its two components. Starting at either pole and following the central "S" curve it can be seen that as one force increases the other complimentary force wanes. Throughout Chinese medical literature there is often described a tripartition of yin and yang. Thus in Figure 1, from bottom to top (right) yang can be seen to progress from minor yang through splendor yang to major yang while from top to bottom (left), it progresses from minor yin through shrinking yin to major yin. It can also be seen centrally that there is some small mount of yin in yang and yang in yin.

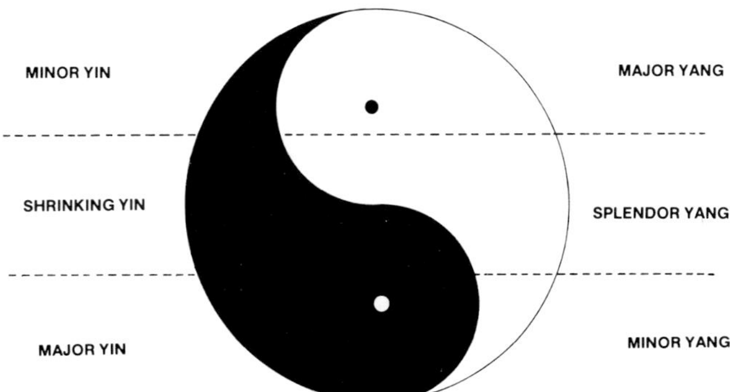

Figure 1. The waxing and waning of Yin and Yang.

In traditional Chinese medicine whole man is the yin/yang. The yin and yang are two life forces which for perfect health must be kept in harmonious balance. Illness occurs when this balance is disturbed. There are yin illnesses and yang illnesses, yin foods and yang foods, herbal medicines to strengthen yin and herbal medicines to strengthen yang. In acupuncture there is, therefore, a major concern with needling procedures to balance yin or yang should either force be deemed weak or in excess.

Second, only in importance to yin and yang was an understanding of the five evolutive phases (wu hsing) often translated "five element theory." This concept was formulated by Tsou Yen who lived between 350-270 B.C. Like much of Chinese medical theory the "wu hsing": fire, earth, metal, wood, and water, refer not to static elements, like a primitive periodic table, but rather energetic qualities that are evolving, expanding and contracting within a time frame.

In our brief attempt here to grasp some fundamentals of a vast and complex metaphysical philosophy, we must conceive of an evolution of forces within the human body that is linked to the changing forces of nature. As we shall see later even the optimal times for treating various diseases is based upon the time of day at which energy is thought to peak within various organ systems.

In keeping with the microcosmic nature of man the doctrine and nature of acupuncture needling must in some ways depend upon not only the hour of the day but as well upon the season of the year and the position of the moon. Table II shows the importance of numerological and astrological concepts for Chinese medicine. It will be noted that this table also indicates clearly the concern of Chinese physicians with the whole man, long predating Western concepts of psychosomatic medicine. Thus, the five evolutive phases are concerned not only with the condition of the physical disease but also with a description of the patient's emotional state as well.

TABLE II

CORRESPONDENCES OF THE FIVE ELEMENTS

	Wood	Fire	Earth	Metal	Water
Solid organ	Liver	Heart	Spleen	Lungs	Kidney
Hollow organ	Gallbladder	Small Intestine	Stomach	Large Instestine	Bladder
Sense	Sight	Words	Taste	Smell	Hearing
Nourishes	Muscles	Circulation	Fat	Skin	Bones
Liquid	Tears	Sweat	Saliva	Mucus	Urine
Smell	Rancid	Scorched	Fragrant	Fleshy	Putrid
Temperament	Depressed	Cyclic	Obsession	Anguish	Fear
Feelings	Anger	Joy	Sympathy	Grief	Anxiety
Flavour	Sour	Bitter	Sweet	Hot	Salt
Sound	Shout	Laugh	Sing	Weep	Groan
Energies	Wind	Heat	Humidity	Dryness	Cold
Season	Spring	Summer	Mid-summer	Autumn	Winter
Colour	Green	Red	Yellow	White	Black
Direction	East	South	Centre	West	North
Development	Birth	Growth	Transformation	Harvest	Store
Cereal	Wheat	Millet	Rye	Rice	Beans
Meat	Chicken	Mutton	Beef	Horse	Pork
Musical note	chio	chih	kung	shang	yu

The basic relationship of the five forces or elements to the functions of nature are displayed in Figure 2. In this diagram it can be seen that spring (east, wood) advances toward summer (south, fire) and hence to autumn (west, metal or air) and on to winter (north, water). This clockwise cycle derived from a central starting point, the earth. In this science of yin/yang cycles it was felt that no life, no growth, nor recovery from illness could come without the cooperation of both heavenly and earthly powers. In this system the five elements operated from the heavens, while six "chhi" or life energies derived from earth. There existed the conviction that man was not isolated from nature, thus cyclic astronomical, meteorological, climactic and epidemiological factors were important for physical processes of health and disease.

The five elements became integrated into yin/yang theory as wood (yang minor), fire (yang major), metal (yin minor) and water (yin major). In ancient sections of the Nei Ching, the fifth or central evolutive phase, earth, is moved to a position between fire and metal where it has since remained in classical tradition (Figure 3). The various organs are believed to relate to or function within this traditional framework.

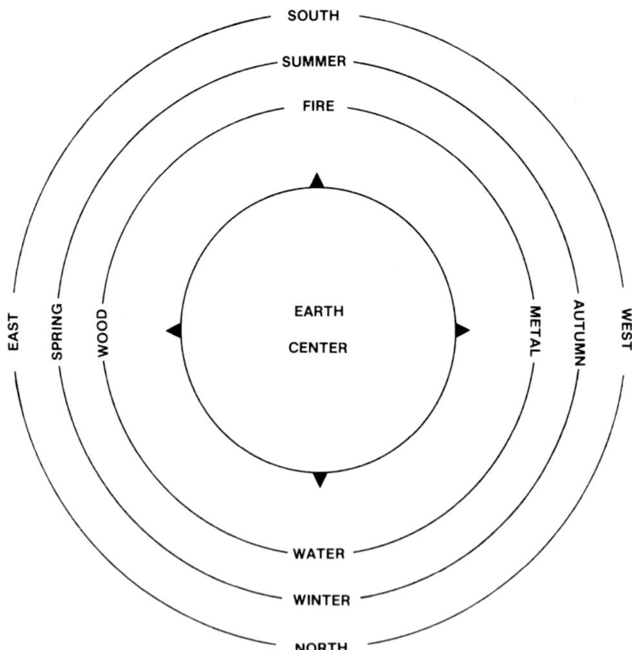

Figure 2. Early designation of the "Five essences" (elements) Wu Hing with earth in the central (center) creative position.

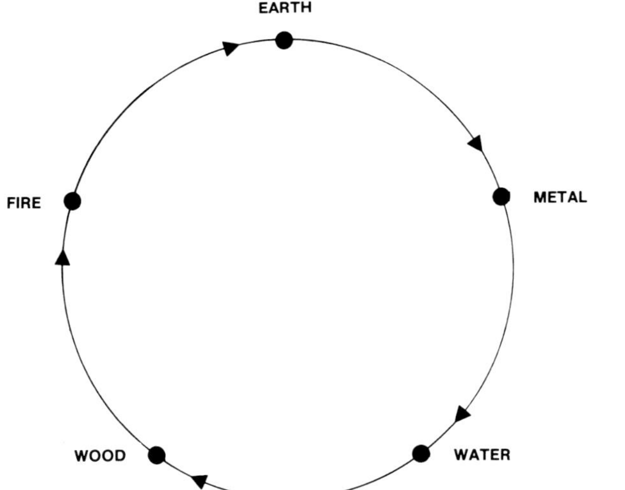

Figure 3. Later designation of the five elements with earth now removed from the center to a position equal with the other four elements.

The so-called "productive sequence," (wu or sheng cycle) conceives of each evolutive phase (element) as the product or "child" (tzo), of each preceding phase (element), which is considered as its "mother" (mu), in clockwise rotation (Figure 4). Similarly, a "checking" sequence (ko cycle), Table III, is described in which each evolutive phase (element), is considered checking the preceding element (counter-clockwise rotation). If the energy at a given position becomes redundant its qualities may overpower the qualities of positions that are functionally connected with it. Under these conditions the checking "ko" function becomes a violation of the "wu" sequence thus producing dysfunction in the corresponding organ or bodily system. Under normal conditions the "productive" and "checking" energetic forces are presumed to act in such fashion as to maintain harmonious balance of function within the organism. In the therapeutic formulations of Chinese medicine, the influence of one organ system upon other organ systems is determined by the relationship of the five evolutive phases to each other.

A consideration of the 12 meridians and the requirement of symmetry in pulse diagnosis seemed to dictate the need for six pairs of organs in relation to the five elements. Thus we find in the completed diagram (Figure 5), that fire has been divided into two parts: the heart prince (heart, small intestine) and the heart minister (pericardium and triple warmer). The triple warmer represents three hypothetical spaces in the abdominal cavity concerned with the creation of energy.

For a time we will leave this discussion of the five evolutive phases to return again after a discussion of Chinese pulse diagnosis.

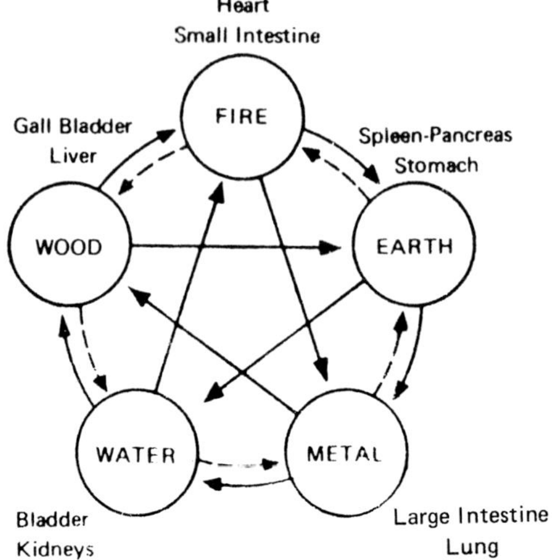

Figure 4. Showing the interaction of the five essences and how they may influence one another. Clockwise rotation is the engendering (strengthening) sheng cycle. Counterclockwise is the overcoming (weakening) ko cycle.

TABLE III

DOCTRINE OF THE FIVE ELEMENTS. "THE LAW OF "WU HING"
Illustrating How These Elements Exercise an Influence One Upon the Other

THE SHENG CYCLE

FIRE engenders EARTH
EARTH engenders METAL
METAL engenders WATER
WATER engenders WOOD
WOOD engenders FIRE

THE KO CYCLE

FIRE overcomes METAL by melting
METAL overcomes WOOD by cutting
WOOD overcomes EARTH by covering
EARTH overcomes WATER by damming
WATER overcomes FIRE by extinguishing

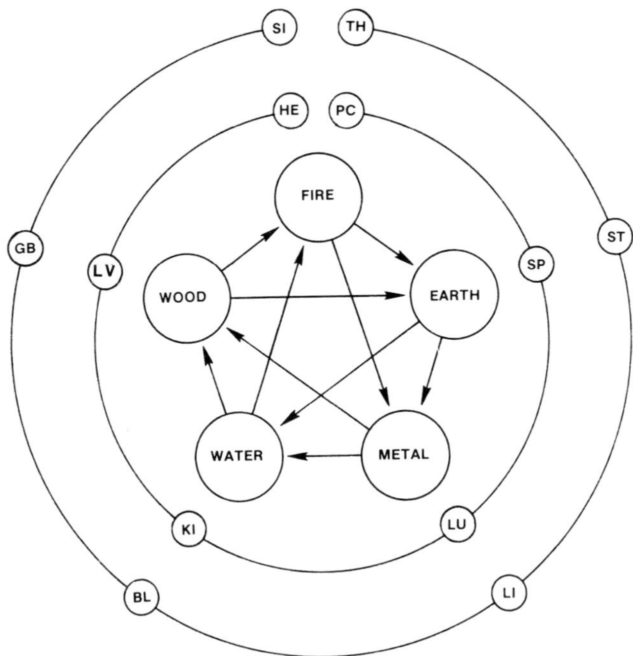

Figure 5. Illustrates the addition of the pericardium (PC) and the triple heaters (TH) to the fire position. This increases the number of organ positions around the five element diagram from 5 to 6 thus permitting concordance with the twelve meridians. Organs shown on the innermost circle are solid (Yin) organs. Those on the outer circle are hollow (Yang) organs.

SPHYGMOLOGY (PULSE DIAGNOSIS)

It is of interest that the Chinese conceived the idea of circulation of the blood 200 years B.C., almost two thousand years before the doctrine of blood circulation was formulated in the West by Harvey, 1628 A.D. (4). The early Chinese physicians held that there were two systems of circulation in the body: one for the blood (mo), concerned with the yin forces. The vaporous life force (chhi) circuit was a yang force circulating in the sinarteries (acupuncture meridian tracts). Both mo and chhi had a dual origin partly from nutritional sources and partly inherited from yin (maternal) and yang (paternal) influences. According to Chinese medicine, under conditions of normal health all parts of the body were supplied with essential elements to replace metabolic loss and to effect repair by the systems of circulation. Any interference with these resulted in disease requiring acupuncture, moxibustion or herbs to restore the proper yin/yang balance.

The Nei-Ching dictated that the pulse should be studied during the early morning hours (3 am to 9 am), when the "ying is immobile and the yang not yet gone from the body." The patient should be fasting with bladder and stomach empty. "At this moment only are blood and energy calm." Such pulse diagnosis was an essential part of Chinese medical practice. It was felt that the radial pulses of the two wrists each provided a reflection of six of the twelve bodily systems indicating the yin/yang balance or the state of health in each (Figure 6).

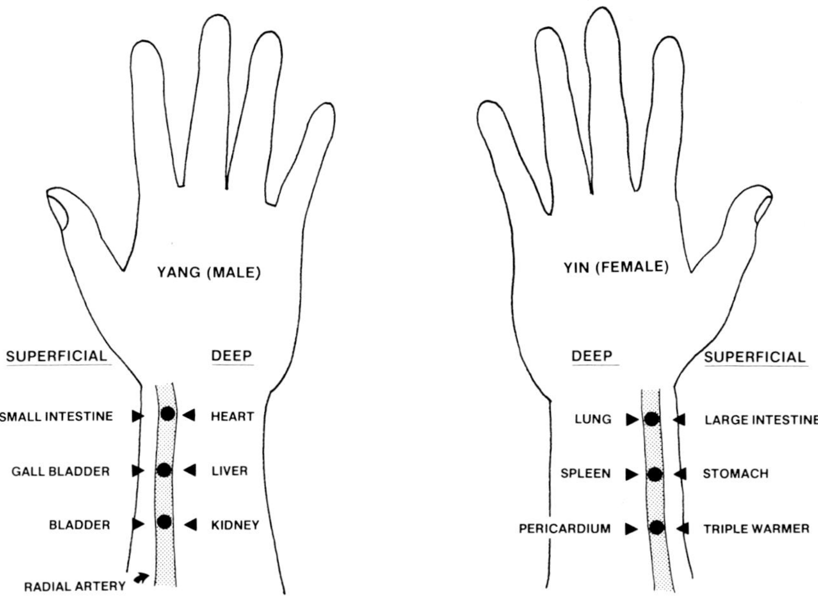

Figure 6. Location of the twelve pulses in relationship to the energy flow to be detected as reflected from the twelve meridians. Interaction between the left and right hand pulses is known as the husband-wife law. Thus the husband may rule the wife but that relationship can be "put in danger" by the wife.

To properly palpate the pulse three fingers, index, middle and ring, were placed upon the radial artery on the radial side of the wrist where the fingers can palpate the artery directly against the radius. The middle finger rests on the bony radial prominence with the index and ring finger palpating the "sun and chhia" sites distally and proximally respectively. There is also a deep and superficial palpation by each of the three fingers. Each pulse is supposed to transmit special information about a specific bodily system. It will be noted that the deep pulses reflect the tsang (solid) organs and the superficial pulses, the fu (hollow) organs. Physicians well trained in pulse diagnosis are claimed to be able to differentiate some 28 qualities of pulse (Table IV). Skilled pulse diagnosticians have the reputation for accurate estimation of prognosis in critically ill cases by means of seven "fatal" pulses, among them, for example, "rolling peas under the finger" (terminal peritonitis), a "feather brushing the cheek" (terminal pulmonary tuberculosis), "movements of a tadpole" (auricular fibrillation), "snapping of a violin's taut string" (hypertensive nephritis), etc. In order to properly assess the pulse the physician must first compose himself in silence, develop his own respiratory rate as normal and count the pulse beats in relation to his own breathing, i.e., four beats of the pulse to each single respiration as a normal baseline.

TABLE IV

QUALITIES OF THE PULSE

Floating	Full	Hollow	Fine
Deep	Long	Wiry (bow-string)	Buried (hidden)
Slow	Short	Leather	Moving
Rapid	Overflowing	Hard	Hasty
Slippery	Minute	Weak-floating	Knotted
Rough	Tight	Weak	Intermittent
Empty	Slowed-down	Scattered	Hurried

Figure 7 is a summary diagram showing as it does the relationship of the twelve pulses to the twelve bodily systems, tsang (yin) and fu (yang) organs and as well to the five elements (evolutive phases). This diagramatic representation depicts an interrelationship which aids in determining which organ system needs to be stimulated or calmed in order to restore an harmonic balance to the total system. If, for example, the pulse representing lung (metal-air) was found deficient one might stimulate spleen (earth), to bring about correction. With the complex interactions shown the same result might be accomplished by acting upon fire (pericardium) or kidney (water). Thus, one can begin to see the multitude of interactions that can be developed within such a metaphysical formulation. The rules for determination of the proper point seem almost endless. It is understandable how a vast number of inconsistencies will be found as one reads the voluminous literature that has accumulated through the centuries.

In considering the causation of illness it was important to recognize the nature and timing of the energy forces circulating within the body. Thus, yin/yang and chhi were felt to circle endlessly making 50 revolutions each day and night of twelve double hours. The order of circulation through the body systems is shown in Figure 8. In addition the ebb and flow of energy in the organ systems followed the clock in such a fashion that energy peaked in each system at a given time of the day or night. There thus appeared times most effective for the treatment of each afflicted organ/system (Figure 9). To ignore this horary cycle was to impair the likelihood of curing the illness.

The theoretical foundations of Chinese medicine thus far summarized form the basis for a therapeutic approach that involves far more than acupuncture. An even larger part of the physician's armamentarium was herbology. A knowledge of the medicinal value of plants was early developed in the Chinese pharmacopia. To each of these herbs was attached, apart from any effect on special organ or systems, the characteristic of yin or yang, thus indicating its ability to either stimulate or sedate given meridian functions.

As Table II illustrates, various colors, sounds, weather, music and specific types of food had their representation of equivalence in the five essences each with specific yin or yang effect. From such a list, changes in life style or diet would be recommended for their beneficial influence upon the life of the individual. This was, indeed, the epitome of holistic medicine, as the advice given for climate, foods, etc., was designed to prevent as well as to cure. It is said that at one period in Chinese medical history the physician was paid only as long as the patient remained well.

With the onset of disease payment ceased, to be resumed only when the physician had accomplished remission from the illness.

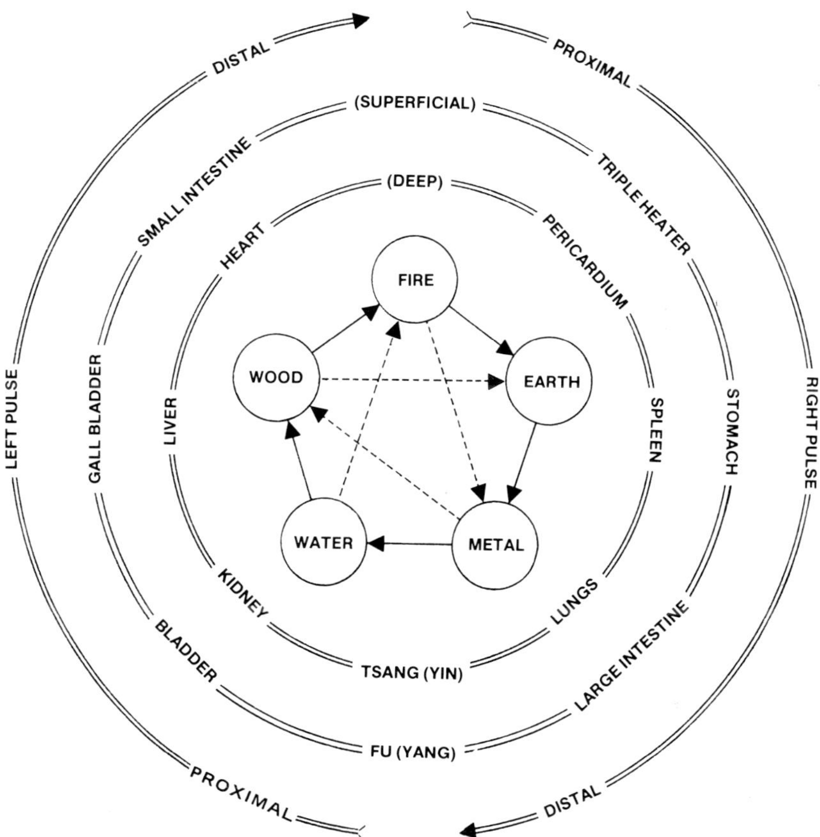

Figure 7. The complete five element diagram showing all twelve organs, the sheng (tonification) and ko (sedating) interactions and as well the correspondence of yin and yang organs to the deep and superficial pulse positions respectively. This diagram displays, in visual form, the basic elements of the great law of Pu-hsieh indicating the placement of needles for the augmentation or dispersal of energy.

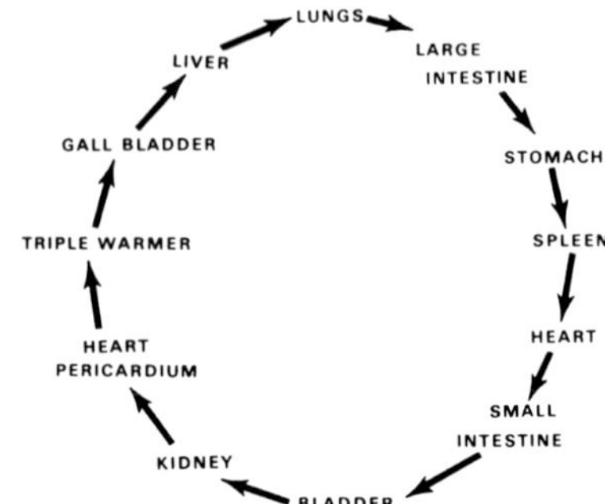

Figure 8. Sequence of energy flow in the twelve meridians.

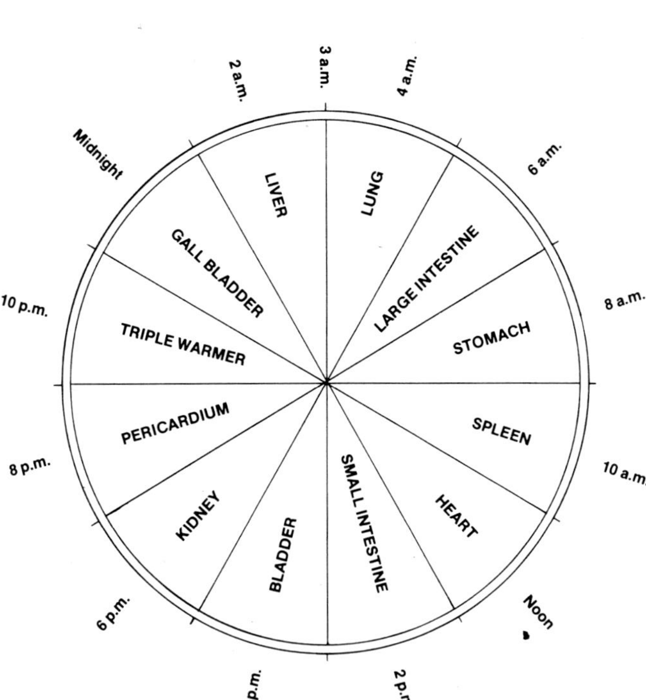

Figure 9. The horary cycle, showing the peaking of energy in the 12 meridians at various designated times in the 24 hour day-night cycle.

Early in the development of Chinese medical history detailed consideration was given as to the specific means for conducting energy through the body. The Huang Ti Nei Ching (Yellow Emperor's Manual of Corporal Medicine), states that in that section known as the Su Wen, blood vessels are to be recognized in the body. In the Ling Shu section it was stated that the ying chhi travels within the blood vessels (mo), while the (yang), wei chhi travels outside of them. It was with this latter system of conduits that the portion of the Nei Ching, known as the Chen Ching (Manual of the Needles) was concerned and laid down the first description of points. These points were located on the main channels (acu-tracts), ching. Each has at least one junction (acu-junction or lo) where it connects with one or more neighboring tracts through short branches (lo-mo). This system of ching-lo (acupuncture tracts or meridians) is an invisible one but was presumed to run in the subcutaneous tissues of the body. Upon the ching-lo (meridians) are located the acupuncture points (hsüeh). The stimulation of these points by needles, pressure, heat, moxibustion or otherwise is felt to influence the flow of chhi through these tracts in such a way as to augment (tonify), or decrease (sedate), and thus reestablish the harmonious yin/yang balance.

There are described twelve major regulatory paired tracts and eight auxillary tracts, two of which are unpaired and regulatory (tu mo and jen mo) and six are connecting. Circulation through the twelve main tracts conforms to the yin/yang cycle. The twelve regular paired meridians are universally used by acupuncturists as "road maps" for the location of acupuncture points. As these acutracts have no real anatomical basis, their use to the acupuncturist can be compared to the use of longitude and latitude familiar to the geographer. The eight auxillary tracts differ in importance and frequency of use by acupuncturists. To-mo and jen-mo are the only ones which have acupuncture points of their own and are regularly used along with the twelve paired meridians. The others interact with the twelve regular tracts and their acupuncture points occur at such junctions and are identical with those of the interacting tracts. One of these, known as the great acu-junction of the spleen is identical with ta-pao (spleen point 21) and has, because of its importance, been at times designated as a 15th regulatory meridian.

Besides the above, there are twelve ching chin, interconnecting neuromuscular tracts. As in ancient Greek anatomy, little distinction was made between tendons, muscles and nerves. The designation of these tracts is similarly unclear. They are thought to pass more superficially than the twelve regular meridians, originate from the tips of the four extremities and pass toward the head but without any relationship to the viscera. They had no specific points but were commonly treated with heat or with cauterizing needles at the site of any muscular pain.

According to ancient Chinese concepts, the acupuncture points were holes in the body for the passage of energy or at least areas where the energy passed close to the surface and could thus be readily influenced. The Chinese term for acupuncture point, "hsüeh," means cave or hollow and, indeed, many of the points are described as a slight depression that is felt in the subcutaneous tissue. During the course of some illnesses certain of these points may become tender to palpation, hence some have been designated "pressure points". At other times they may be felt as fibrositic nodules beneath the skin coincident with the modern concept of "trigger points". The number of recognized acupuncture points has varied over time and with different authors. The named points on the regularly used 14 channels total 361. Except for the 51 points of the midline channels, they are mirror-images, duplicated on both sides of the body bringing the total to 671 points. Figures 10 a-n are charts of the 14 major meridians containing all 671 acupuncture points. Table V lists the points by meridian with their Chinese names. Table VI gives common abbreviations of these meridians as used by different authors. In addition, there are, as of this writing, some 63 extra meridian points (chhi hsüeh), commonly used which are not located on any of the meridians. Another 168 acu-points have been described on the ear called "fan ying tien" and each related to some particular viscera or portion on the body surface. Figure 11 shows a plastic mannequin such as used in the People's Republic of China today in teaching acupuncture meridians and points.

While the above are the commonly accepted points there are, in addition, "private" points discussed and used in their practice by individual acupuncturists. With the growth of acupuncture analgesia for surgery, trial and error experimentation has yielded other points that seem useful for operative procedures and thus today the number of points used in acupuncture may well be over 1000.

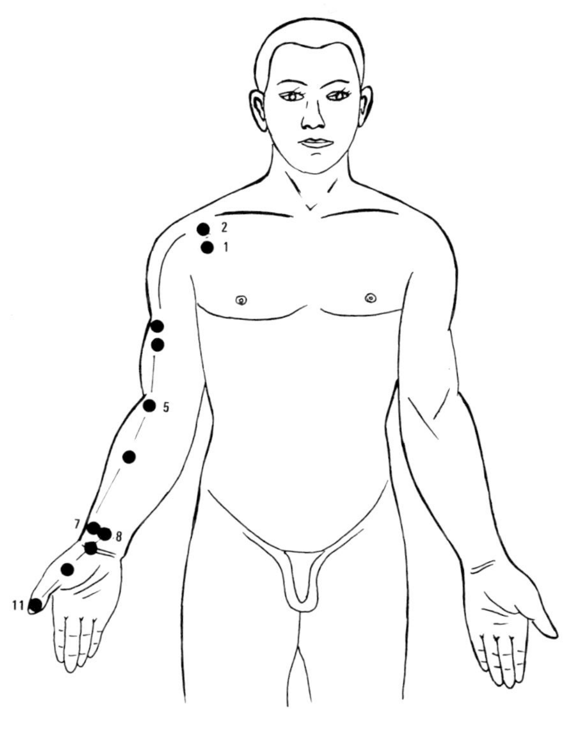

LUNG MERIDIAN

Figure 10. Diagram of the traditional meridians with their acupuncture points.

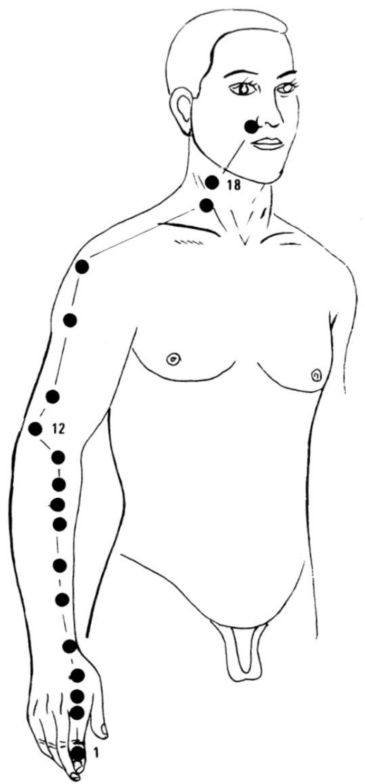

LARGE INTESTINE MERIDIAN

Figure 10 B.

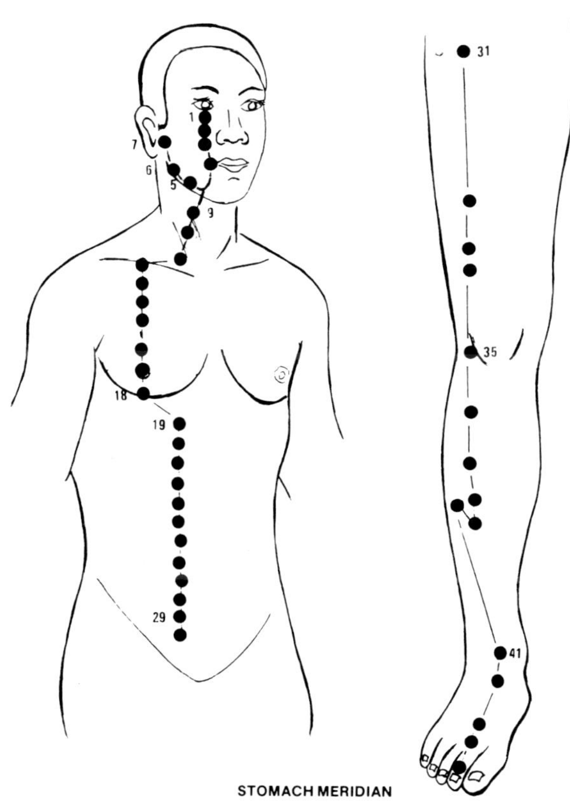

STOMACH MERIDIAN

Figure 10 C.

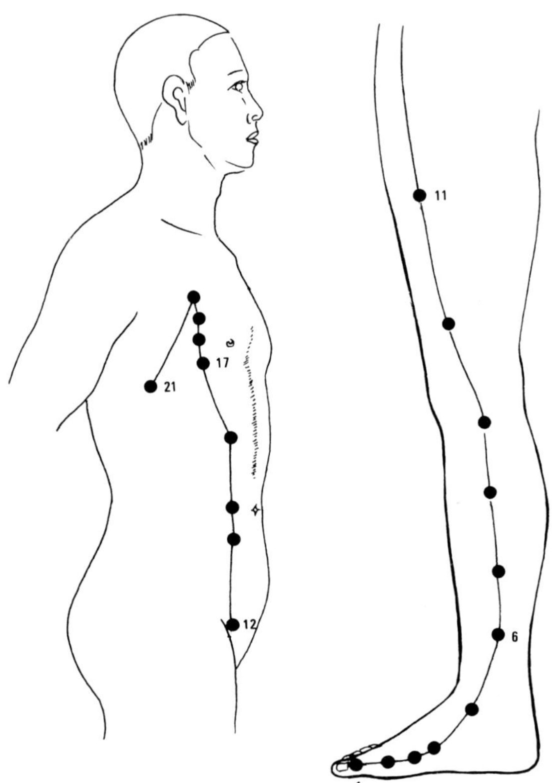

SPLEEN MERIDIAN

Figure 10 D.

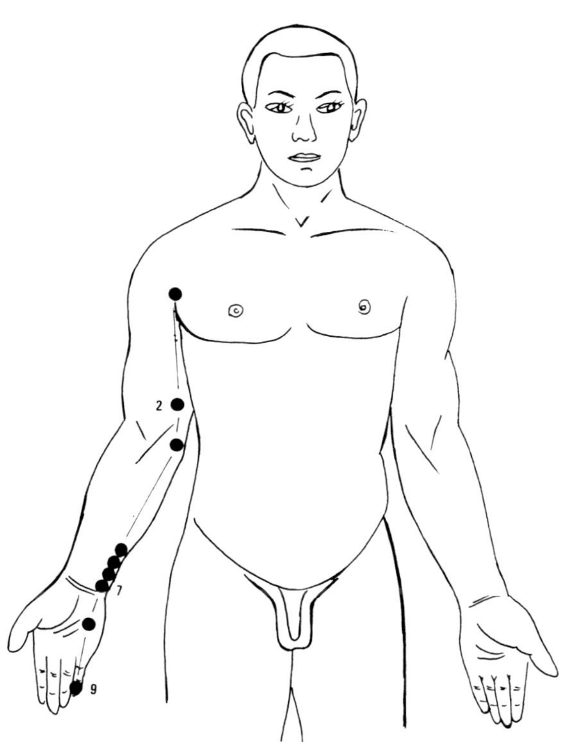

HEART MERIDIAN
Figure 10 E.

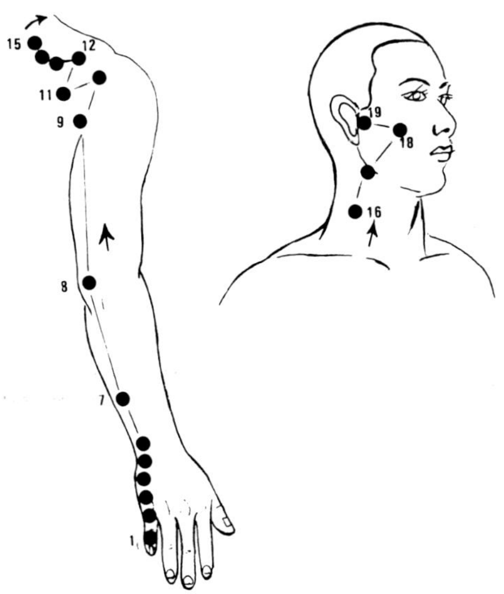

SMALL INTESTINE MERIDIAN

Figure 10 F.

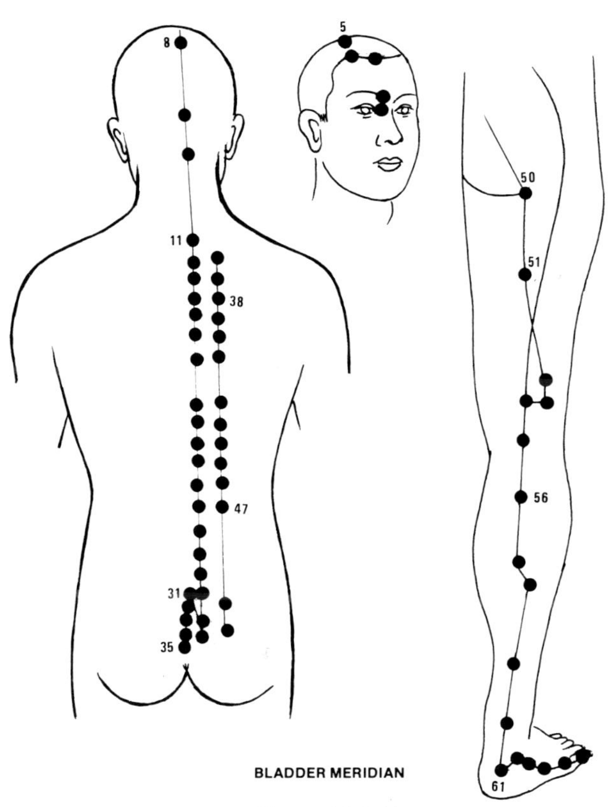

BLADDER MERIDIAN

Figure 10 G.

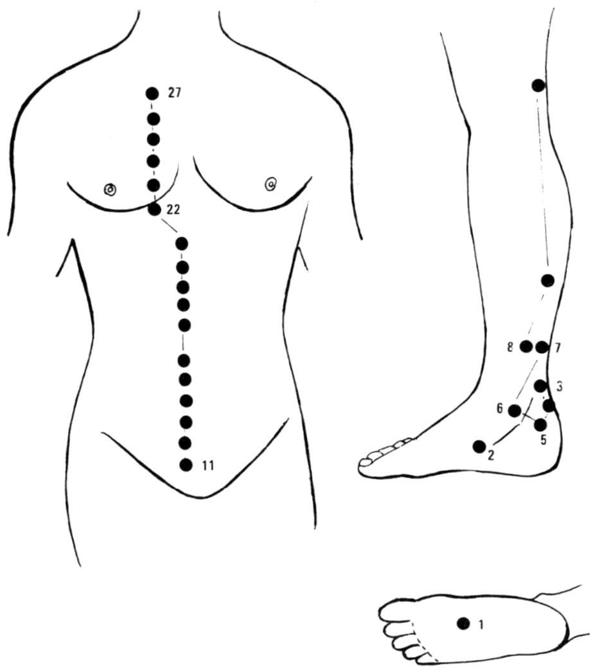

KIDNEY MERIDIAN

Figure 10 H.

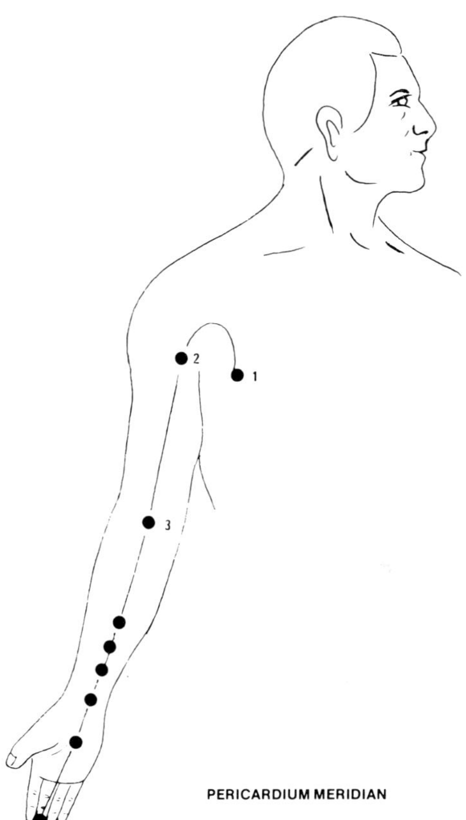

Figure 10 I.

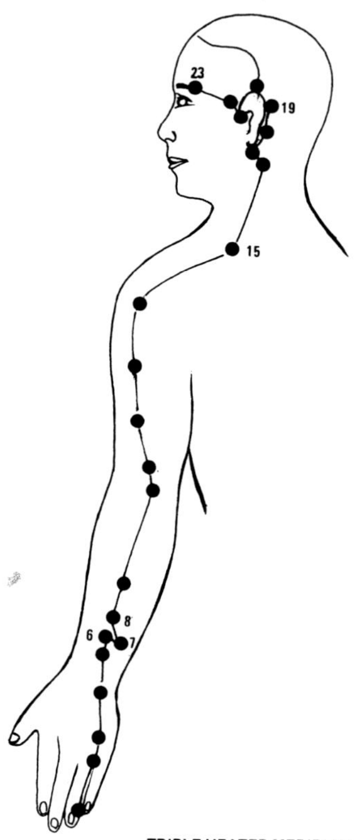

Figure 10 J.

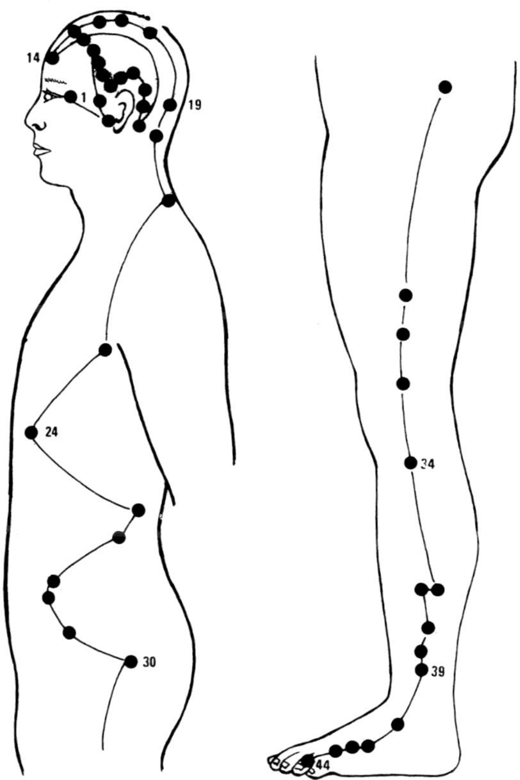

GALL BLADDER MERIDIAN

Figure 10 K.

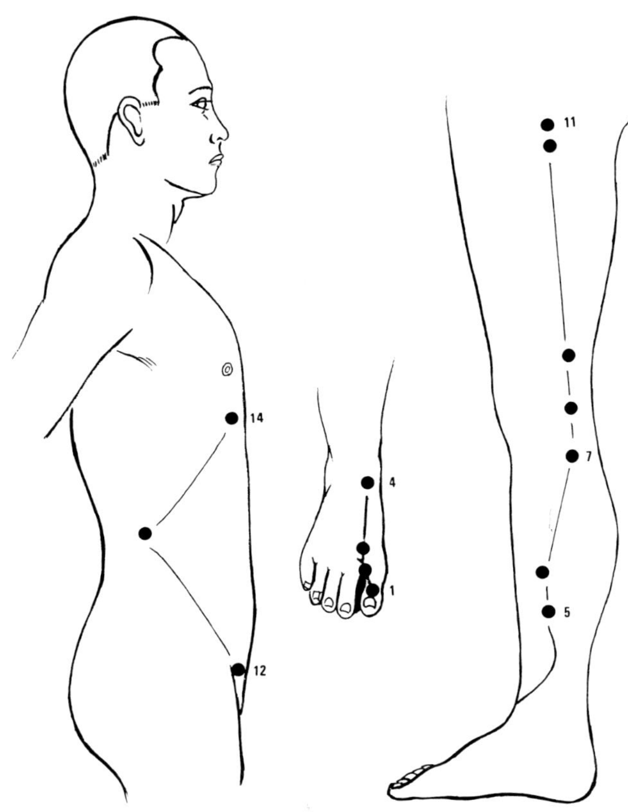

LIVER MERIDIAN

Figure 10 L.

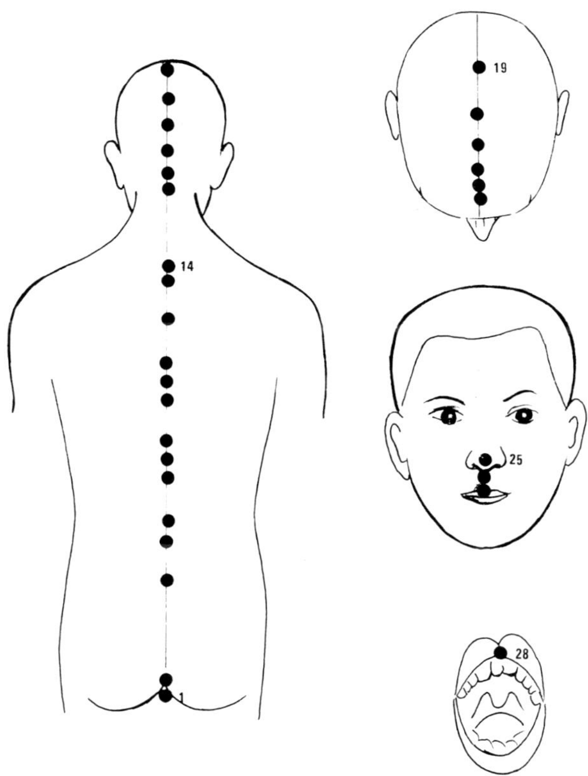

GOVERNING VESSEL MERIDIAN

Figure 10 M.

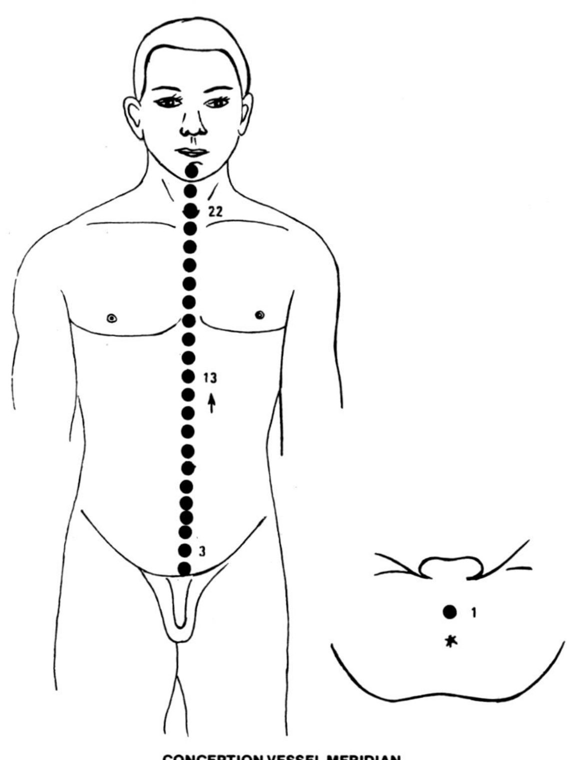

CONCEPTION VESSEL MERIDIAN

Figure 10 N.

TABLE V

ACUPUNCTURE POINTS OF THE FOURTEEN MAIN MERIDIANS

LUNG

1	Chung-fu	中府
2	Yün-mên	雲門
3	Thien-fu	天府
4	Hsia-pai	俠白
5	Chhih-tsê	尺澤
6	Khung-tsui	孔最
7	Lieh-chhüeh	列缺
8	Ching-chhü	經渠
9	Thai-yuan	太淵
10	Yü-chi	魚際
11	Shao-shang	少商

LARGE INTESTINE

1	Shang-yang	商陽
2	Erh-chien	二間
3	San-chien	三間
4	Ho-ku	合谷
5	Yang-chhi	陽谿
6	Phien-li	偏歷
7	Wên-liu	溫溜
8	Hsia-lien	下廉
9	Shang-lien	上廉
10	San-li	三里
11	Chhü-chhih	曲池
12	Chou-liao	肘髎
13	Wu-li	五里
14	Pei-nao	臂臑
15	Chien-yung	肩髃
16	Chü-ku	巨骨
17	Thien-ting	天鼎
18	Fu-thu	扶突
19	Ho-liao	禾髎
20	Ying-hsiang	迎香

STOMACH

1	Thou-wei	頭維
2	Hsia-kuan	下關
3	Chia-chhê[d]	頰車
4	Chhêng-chhi	承泣
5	Ssu-pai	四白
6	Chü-liao	巨髎
7	Ti-tshang	地倉
8	Ta-ying	大迎
9	Jen-ying	人迎
10	Shui-thu	水突
11	Chhi-shê	氣舍
12	Chhüeh-phên	缺盆
13	Chhi-hu	氣戶
14	Khu-fang	庫房
15	Wu-i	屋翳
16	Ying-chhuang	膺窗
17	Ju-chung	乳中
18	Ju-kên	乳根
19	Pu-jung	不容
20	Chhêng-man	承滿
21	Liang-mên	梁門
22	Kuan-mên	關門
23	Thai-i	太乙
24	Hua-jo-mên	滑肉門
25	Thien-shu	天樞
26	Wai-ling	外陵
27	Ta-chü	大巨
28	Shui-tao	水道
29	Kuei-lai	歸來
30	Chhi-chhung	氣衝
31	Phi-kuan	髀關
32	Fu-thu	伏兔
33	Yin-shih	陰市
34	Liang-chhiu	梁邱
35	Tu-pi	犢鼻
36	San-li	三里
37	Shang-chü-hsü	上巨虛
38	Thiao-khou	條口
39	Hsia-chü-hsü	下巨虛
40	Fêng-lung	豐隆
41	Chieh-chhi	解谿
42	Chhung-yang	衝陽
43	Hsien-ku	陷谷
44	Nei-thing	內庭
45	Li-tui	厲兌

SPLEEN

1	Yin-pai	隱白
2	Ta-tu	大都
3	Thai-pai	太白
4	Kung-sun	公孫
5	Shang-chhiu	商邱
6	San-yin-chiao	三陰交
7	Lou-ku	漏谷
8	Ti-chi	地機
9	Yin-ling-chhüan	陰陵泉
10	Hsüeh-hai	血海
11	Chi-mên	箕門
12	Chhung-mên	衝門
13	Fu-shê	府舍
14	Fu-chieh	腹結
15	Ta-hêng	大橫
16	Fu-ai	腹哀
17	Shih-tou	食竇
18	Thien-chhi	天谿
19	Hsiung-hsiang	胸鄉

TABLE V (Cont'd.)

ACUPUNCTURE POINTS OF THE FOURTEEN MAIN MERIDIANS

No.	Name	Chinese
20	Chou-jung	周榮
21	Ta-pao	大包

HEART

No.	Name	Chinese
1	Chi-chhüan	極泉
2	Chhing-ling	青靈
3	Shao-hai	少海
4	Ling-tao	靈道
5	Thung-li	通里
6	Yin-chhi	陰郄
7	Shen-mên	神門
8	Shao-fu	少府
9	Shao-chhung	少衝

SMALL INTESTINE

No.	Name	Chinese
1	Shao-tsê	少澤
2	Chhien-ku	前谷
3	Hou-chhi	後谿
4	Wan-ku	腕骨
5	Yang-ku	陽谷
6	Yang-lao	養老
7	Chih-chêng	支正
8	Hsiao-hai	小海
9	Chien-chên	肩貞
10	Nao-shu	臑兪
11	Thien-tsung	天宗
12	Ping-fêng	秉風
13	Chhü-yuan	曲垣
14	Chien-wai-shu	肩外兪
15	Chien-chung-shu	肩中兪
16	Thien-chuang	天窗
17	Thien-jung	天容
18	Chhüan-liao	顴髎
19	Thing-kung	聽宮

BLADDER

No.	Name	Chinese
1	Ching-ming	睛明
2	Tshuan-chu	攢竹
3	Mei-chhung	眉衝
4	Chhü-chhai	曲差
5	Wu-chhu	五處
6	Chhêng-kuang	承光
7	Thung-thien	通天
8	Lo-chhio	絡却
9	Yü-chen	玉枕
10	Thien-chu	天柱
11	Ta-chu	大杼
12	Fêng-mên	風門
13	Fei-shu	肺兪
14	Chüeh-yin-shu	厥陰兪
15	Hsin-shu	心兪
16	Tu-shu	督兪
17	Ko-shu	膈兪
18	Kan-shu	肝兪
19	Tan-shu	膽兪
20	Phi-shu	脾兪
21	Wei-shu	胃兪
22	San-chiao-shu	三焦兪
23	Shen-shu	腎兪
24	Chhi-hai-shu	氣海兪
25	Ta-chhang-shu	大腸兪
26	Kuan-yuan-shu	關元兪
27	Hsiao-chhang-shu	小腸兪
28	Phang-kuang-shu	膀胱兪
29	Chung-lü-shu	中膂兪
30	Pai-huan-shu	白環兪
31	Shang-liao	上髎
32	Tzhu-liao	次髎
33	Chung-liao	中髎
34	Hsia-liao	下髎
35	Hui-yang	會陽
36	Fu-fên	附分
37	Pho-hu	魄戶
38	Kao-huang	膏肓
39	Shen-thang	神堂
40	I-hsi	譩譆
41	Ko-kuan	膈關
42	Hun-mên	魂門
43	Yang-kang	陽綱
44	I-shê	意舍
45	Wei-tshang	胃倉
46	Huang-mên	肓門
47	Chih-shih	志室
48	Pao-huang	胞肓
49	Chih-pien	秩邊
50	Chhêng-fu	承扶
51	Yin-mên	殷門
52	Fou-chhi	浮郄
53	Wei-yang	委陽
54	Wei-chung	委中
55	Chhêng-chin	承筋
56	Ho-yang	合陽
57	Chhêng-shan	承山
58	Fei-yang	飛陽
59	Fu-yang	付陽
60	Khun-lun	崑崙
61	Phu-shen	僕參
62	Shen-mo	申脉
63	Chin-mên	金門
64	Ching-ku	京骨
65	Shu-ku	束骨

TABLE V (Cont'd.)
ACUPUNCTURE POINTS OF THE FOURTEEN MAIN MERIDIANS

No.	Point	Chinese
66	Thung-ku	通谷
67	Chih-yin	至陰

KIDNEY

No.	Point	Chinese
1	Yung-chhüan	湧泉
2	Jan-ku	然谷
3	Thai-chhi	太谿
4	Ta-chung	大鍾
5	Shui-chhüan	水泉
6	Chao-hai	照海
7	Fu-liu	復溜
8	Chiao-hsin	交信
9	Chu-pin	築賓
10	Yin-ku	陰谷
11	Hêng-ku	橫骨
12	Ta-ho	大赫
13	Chhi-hsüeh	氣穴
14	Ssu-man	四滿
15	Chung-chu	中注
16	Huang-shu	肓兪
17	Shang-chhü	商曲
18	Shih-kuan	石關
19	Yin-tu	陰都
20	Thung-ku	通谷
21	Yu-mên	幽門
22	Pu-lang	步廊
23	Shen-fêng	神封
24	Ling-hsü	靈墟
25	Shen-tsang	神藏
26	Yü-chung	彧中
27	Shu-fu	兪府

PERICARDIUM

No.	Point	Chinese
1	Thien-chhih	天池
2	Thien-chhüan	天泉
3	Chhü-tsê	曲澤
4	Chhi-mên	郄門
5	Chien-shih	間使
6	Nei-kuan	內關
7	Ta-ling	大陵
8	Lao-kung	勞宮
9	Chung-chhung	中衝

TRIPLE HEATER

No.	Point	Chinese
1	Kuan-chhung	關衝
2	I-mên	液門
3	Chung-chu	中渚
4	Yang-chhih	陽池
5	Wai-kuan	外關
6	Chih-kou	支溝
7	Hui-tsung	會宗
8	San-yang-lo	三陽絡
9	Ssu-tu	四瀆
10	Thien-ching	天井
11	Chhing-lêng-yuan	清冷淵
12	Hsiao-lo	消濼
13	Nao-hui	臑會
14	Chien-chiao	肩髎
15	Thien-liao	天髎
16	Thien-yu	天牖
17	I-fêng	翳風
18	Chhi-mo	瘈脈
19	Lu-hsi	顱息
20	Chio-sun	角孫
21	Ssu-chu-khung	絲竹空
22	Ho-liao	和髎
23	Erh-mên	耳門

GALL BLADDER

No.	Point	Chinese
1	Thung-tzu-liao	瞳子髎
2	Thing-hui	聽會
3	Kho-chu-jen	客主人
4	Han-yen	頷厭
5	Hsüan-lu	懸顱
6	Hsüan-li	懸釐
7	Chhü-ping	曲鬢
8	Shuai-ku	率谷
9	Pên-shen	本神
10	Yang-pai	陽白
11	Lin-chhi	臨泣
12	Mu-chuang	目窗
13	Chhiao-yin	竅陰
14	Chhêng-ling	承靈
15	Thien-chhung	天衝
16	Fou-pai	浮白
17	Wan-ku	完骨
18	Chêng-ying	正營
19	Nao-khung	腦空
20	Fêng-chhih	風池
21	Chien-ching	肩井
22	Yuan-i	淵液
23	Chê-chin	輒筋
24	Jih-yüeh	日月

TABLE V (Cont'd.)

ACUPUNCTURE POINTS OF THE FOURTEEN MAIN MERIDIANS

No.	Point	Chinese
25	Ching-mên	京門
26	Tai-mo	帶脈
27	Wu-shu	五樞
28	Wei-tao	維道
29	Chü-liao	居髎
30	Huan-thiao	環跳
31	Fêng-shih	風市
32	Chung-tu	中瀆
33	Yang-kuan	陽關
34	Yang-ling-chhüan	陽陵泉
35	Yang-chiao	陽交
36	Wai-chhiu	外丘
37	Kuang-ming	光明
38	Yang-fu	陽輔
39	Hsüan-chung	懸鍾
40	Chhiu-hsü	丘墟
41	Tsu-lin-chhi	足臨泣
42	Ti-wu-hui	地五會
43	Hsia-chhi	俠谿
44	Tsu-chhiao-yin	足竅陰
	LIVER	
1	Ta-tun	大敦
2	Hsing-chien	行間
3	Thai-chhung	太衝
4	Chung-fêng	中封
5	Li-kou	蠡溝
6	Chung-tu	中都
7	Hsi-kuan	膝關
8	Chhü-chhüan	曲泉
9	Yin-pao	陰包
10	Wu-li	五里
11	Yin-lien	陰廉
12	Chi-mo	急脈
13	Chang-mên	章門
14	Chhi-mên	期門
	GOVERNING VESSEL	
1	Chhang-chhiang	長強
2	Yao-shu	腰兪
3	Yang-kuan	陽關
4	Ming-mên	命門
5	Hsüan-shu	懸樞
6	Chi-chung	脊中
7	Chin-so	筋縮
8	Chih-yang	至陽
9	Ling-thai	靈臺
10	Shen-tao	神道
11	Shen-chu	身柱
12	Hsiung-tao	胸道
13	Ta-chhui	大椎
14	Ya-mên	瘂門
15	Fêng-fu	風府
16	Nao-hu	腦戶
17	Chhiang-chien	強間
18	Hou-ting	後頂
19	Pai-hui	百會
20	Chhien-ting	前頂
21	Hsing-hui	顖會
22	Shang-hsing	上星
23	Shen-thing	神庭
24	Su-liao	素髎
25	Shui-kou	水溝
26	Tui-tuan	兌端
27	Yin-chiao	齦交
	CONCEPTION VESSEL	
1	Hui-yin	會陰
2	Chhü-ku	曲骨
3	Chung-chi	中極
4	Kuan-yuan	關元
5	Shih-mên	石門
6	Chhi-hai	氣海
7	Yin-chiao	陰交
8	Shen-chhüeh	神闕
9	Shui-fên	水分
10	Hsiz-kuan	下脘
11	Chien-li	建里
12	Chung-kuan	中脘
13	Shang-kuan	上脘
14	Chü-chhüeh	巨闕
15	Chiu-wei	鳩尾
16	Chung-thing	中庭
17	Shan-chung	膻中
18	Yü-thang	玉堂
19	Tzu-kung	紫宮
20	Hua-kai	華蓋
21	Hsüan-chi	璇璣
22	Thien-thu	天突
23	Lien-chhüan	廉泉
24	Chhêng-chiang	承漿

TABLE VI

MERIDIAN ABBREVIATIONS AS USED BY SEVERAL AUTHORS

	SOURCE								
MERIDIAN	Needham and Lu	Mann	Several French Authors	Wu Wei Ping	Nat. Acup. Res. Society	Choi	Porkert	Shanghai Traditional Institute	Ulett
I Lung (Pulmonic)	P	L	P	LU	LU	L	P	P	LU
II Large Intestine (Crasso-Intestinal Colon)	IG	Li	GI	CO	LI	LI	IC	IC	LI
III Stomach (Gastric)	V	S	E	ST	STO	S	S	G	ST
IV Spleen (Pancreas) (Lienic)	LP	Sp	RP	SP	SPL	Sp	L	LP	SP
V Heart (Cardiac)	C	H	C	HE	H	H	C	C	HE
VI Small Intestine (Tenu-Intestinal)	IT	Si	IG	SI	SI	SI	IT	IT	SI
VII Bladder (Vesical)	VU	B	V	BL	B	B	V	VU	BL
VIII Kidney (Reno-Seminal)	R	K	R	KI	K	K	R	R	KI
IX Pericardium (Envelope of Heart) (Heart Constrictor) (Circulation - Sex)	HC	P	MCS	HC	P	P	PC	PC	PC
X Tri-Heater (Triple Warmer) (Triple Scorcher) (TN-Coctive)	SC	T	TR	TH	TH	TS	T	T	TH
XI Gall Bladder (Felleic)	VF	G	VB	GB	GB	GB	F	VF	GB
XII Liver (Hepatic)	H	Liv	F	LI	LV	LIV	H	H	LV
XIII Governing Vessel (Dorsal Meridian Regulative) Tuo mo	TM	Gv	Vg	VG	G	GV	Rg	TM	GV
XIV Conception Vessel (Ventral Meridian Regulative) Jen mo	JM	Cv	Vc	VC	C	Cv	Rs	JM	CV

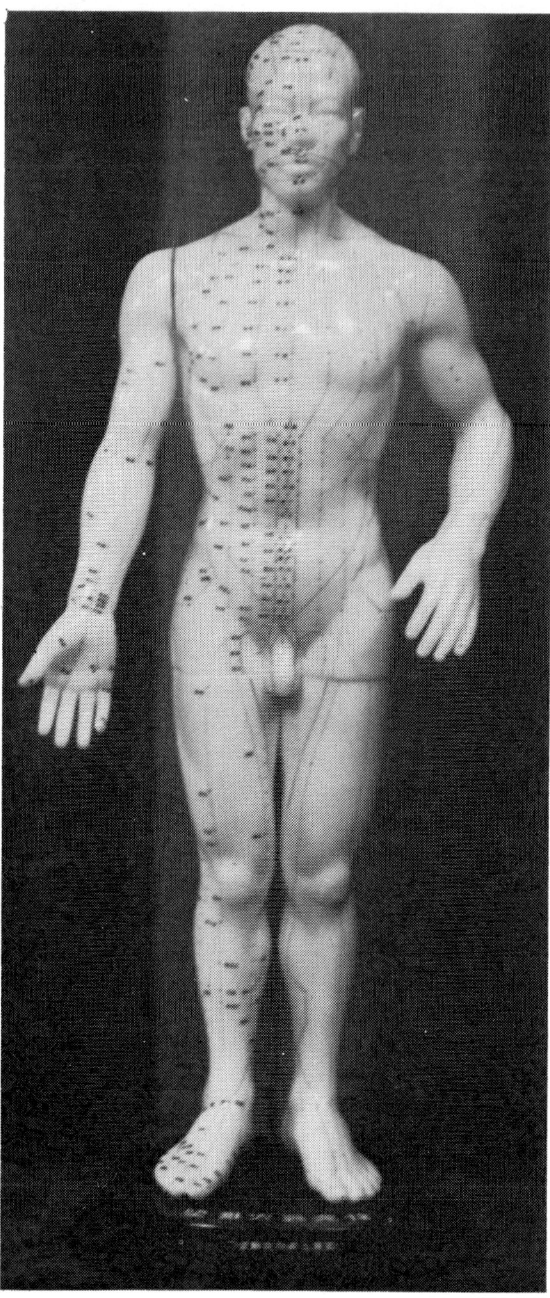

Figure 11. Plastic mannequin used for teaching traditional acupuncture points.

Each of these acupuncture points is carefully described in terms of its surface anatomical location. Their identification was dependent upon local landmarks of the body, such as bony tubercles, the nipples, depressions in muscular structures, etc. For the location of points away from such landmarks a system of body measurements was developed. In order to allow for differences in body size a unit of self measurement known as the "chun," "pouce" or "body inch" was developed. This was the distance between two folds of the middle phalanx of the middle finger in a bent position (Figure 12). This body inch was subdivided into 10 lesser units termed "fen." Each point has a designated usefulness for the treatment of some type of illness or symptom. Descriptions of these may be found in the many texts on the subject. While most authors agree very well on the location of points there is considerable variance as to their therapeutic value.

ONE CHUN

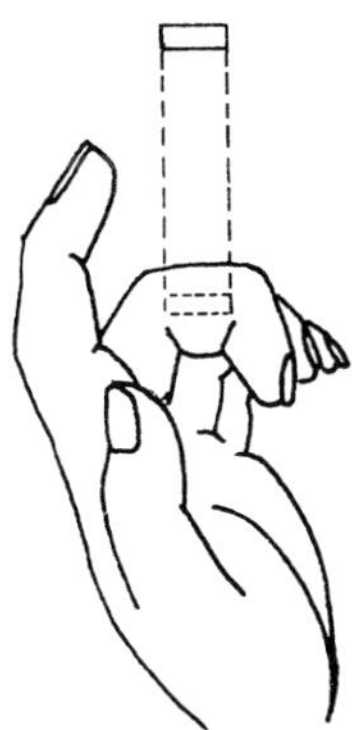

Figure 12. "Chun" acupuncture unit of measurement.

Some classes of points are commonly referred to as having specific therapeutic application (Table VII). These include: points having strong influence over the relationship of meridians to organ functions: tsing points (tips of fingers and toes), yung points (base of fingers and toes), yu points (hands and feet), ching points (wrists and ankles) and wo points (elbows and knees).

Points of Origin: (Source or yuan points): These occur where the organ is said to give its energy to the corresponding meridian. These are useful in treating dysfunction of that specific organ system.

Points of Anastamosis: (lo points): Here is where the yin and yang meridians communicate. Points of contact are between the tsang and fu organs.

Points of Accumulation: (hsi points): Useful in treating chronic disease. Points where the energy is thought to accumulate.

Points of Relationship Between Ventral and Dorsal Meridians: Mo points and shu points. These are located respectively on the ventral and dorsal aspects of the body, close to the visceral organs upon which they are felt to have a mutual influence.

Points of Conveyance: (wei points): These points are felt to be useful in the treatment of illness of different types of tissue, viscera and energy as follows:

Tsang (yin viscera) LI-13
Fu (yang viscera) CV-12
Chhi (energy) CV-17
Blood BL-17
Bone BL-11
Bone marrow GB-39
Tendons-muscle GB-34
Meridians LU-9

Special points: Connecting points between the twelve paired and eight auxillary meridians. These are thought to have special stimulating influence each over its own meridian as well to spread its effect widely through the connecting meridian.

TABLE VII

DESIGNATION OF SOME ACUPUNCTURE POINTS BELIEVED TO HAVE SPECIFIC THERAPEUTIC APPLICATION

SIXTY POINTS OF COMMAND

GB	TH	BL	SI	ST	LI				Liv	HC	KI	HT	SP	LU
44	1	67	1	45	1	METAL	TSING (energy emerging) tips fingers and toes	WOOD	1	9	1	9	1	11
43	2	66	2	44	2	WATER	YUNG (energy streaming) base fingers and toes	FIRE	2	8	2	8	2	10
41	3	65	3	43	3	WOOD	YU (energy filling) knees and feet	EARTH	3	7	3	7	3	9
38	6	60	5	41	5	FIRE	CHING (energy passing) wrists and knees	METAL	4	5	7	4	5	8
34	10	54	8	36	11	EARTH	HO (energy meeting) elbows and knees	WATER	8	3	10	3	9	5
40	4	64	4	42	4		YUAN (origin) organ transmits energy to meridian		3	7	3-5	7	3	9
37	5	58	7	40	6		LO (Le) (communication) where yin meets yang		5	6	4	5	4	7
36	7	63	6	34	7		HSI (accumulation) where energy accumulates		6	4	4	6	8	6
41	6	66	5	36	1		HORARY (hourly) where energy is at maximum		1	8	10	8	3	8
1	1	1	1	1	4		ENTRY		1	1	1	1	1	1
41	23	67	19	41	20		EXIT		14	8	22	9	21	7
Liv 14	VC 15	GB 25	VC 14	Liv 13	LU 1		ALARM-REFLEX PTS.		GB 23 24	VC 5-7 12-17	VC 3	VC 4	VC 12	ST 25

EAR ACUPUNCTURE THERAPY (AURICULOTHERAPY)

The ear has long been implicated in traditional acupuncture. Several chapters of the Nei Ching make reference to the six yang meridians as passing through the ear. Later writings state that all twelve meridians are joined in the ear. The Nei Ching also refers to the ear as useful in diagnosing afflictions of the kidney. From the 5th century A.D., acupuncture of the ear was mentioned in the treatment of many diseases. In 1957, the French physician and acupuncturist, Paul Nogier, reported studies relating the ear to other parts of the body. He teachings have served to popularize the subspecialty of auriculotherapy (5). Today ear acupuncture has increased throughout the world and it is often used as a sole or supplementary treatment for some 60-70 types of ailment. In China, ear points are often stimulated in combination with body points or are used alone in acupuncture analgesia for surgery. Currently 168 ear points have been identified, each corresponding to a different part of the body. Some of these are shown in Figure 13.

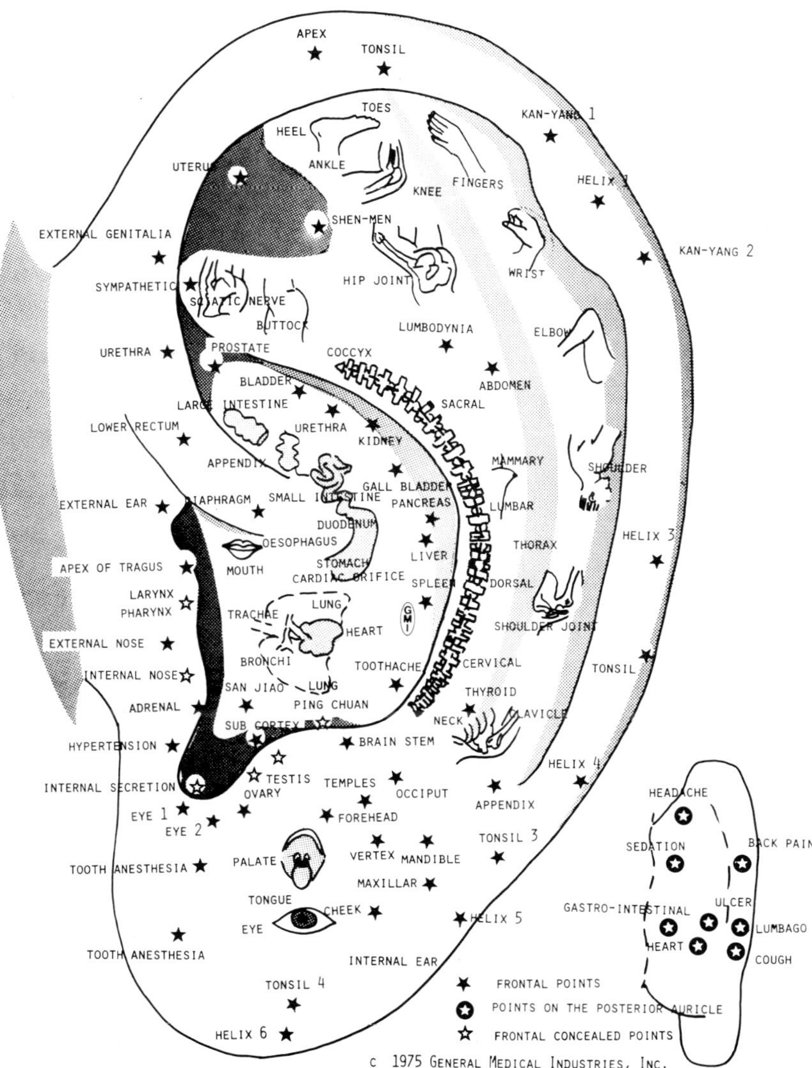

Figure 13. Theorized correspondence between designated points on the auricle and regions of body anatomy. It is important to note that the major body organs as supplied by the autonomic nervous system lie within the concha of the ear, an area supplied by the vagus nerve.

The distribution of points in the ear is such that the head and neck are located in the lower portion with the remainder of the body upward and in such fashion that it has been likened to an upside down embryo (Figure 14).

According to Nogier, when a certain part of the body undergoes a pathological change, pressure pain points (reaction points) or areas of visible discoloration, scales, etc., appear in the corresponding part of the ear. When these points of reference are pressed with a fine, blunt instrument, the patient may cry out with pain. Such areas are treated with pressure, acupuncture or electrical stimulation in order to bring about relief from pain or symptoms in the corresponding part of the body.

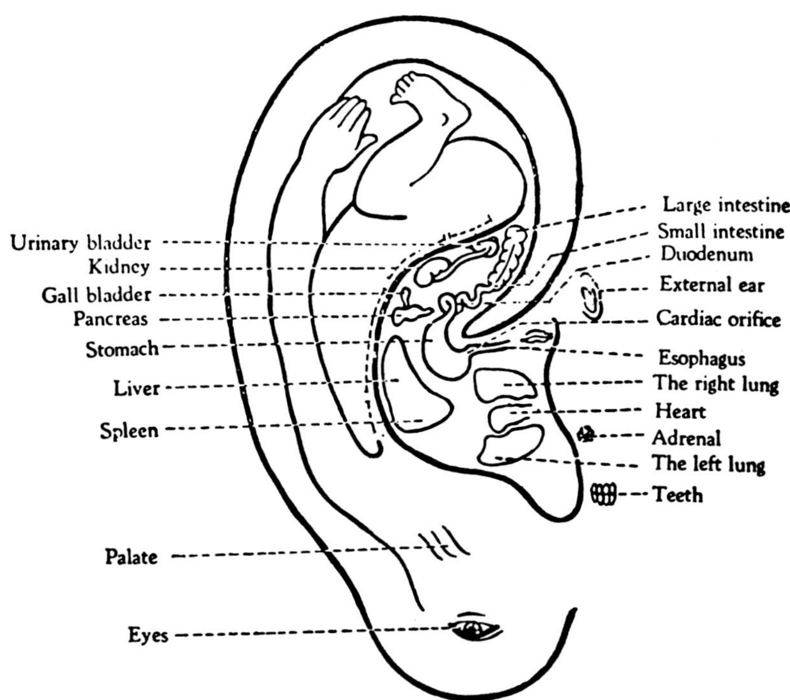

Figure 14. Corresponding anatomical representation of body areas to ear points resembling an embryo "upside down" within the auricle. From Lu, Gwei-Djen and Needham, J.: *Celestial Lancets.* Cambridge University Press, 1980, p. 427.

Wen (6), of Hong Kong, used electrical stimulation of the ear for the treatment of addiction. It is reported (7), that addiction to different drugs requires different frequencies of stimulation. Other addictive ailments, obesity, smoking, etc., have been so treated with small press needles, staples and beads that are inserted or sewed in place and left for varying lengths of time. The patient is instructed to press upon the bead or staple in order to self-stimulate these acupuncture points. It is of interest that the ear is innervated by five major nerves. Most important of all is the fact that the concha of the ear is innervated by the vagus nerve. The concha of the ear is the only place that the vagus can be reached on the surface of the body. This may well explain its effectiveness in treating a wide variety of body ailments as well as its use in the treatment of anxiety and the symptoms of drug withdrawal in addicts where it functions through a calming of the visceral functions by stimulation of the parasympathetic division of the autonomic nervous system.

OTHER RELATED ACUPUNCTURE THERAPIES (8)

Moxibustion

This consists of the application of heat to acupuncture points. Moxa is a punk-like substance made from the herb, Artemesia Vulgaris (Mugwort). The best leaves of the plant were collected during the 5th month of the Chinese calendar, then thoroughly dried and ground to a white powder. This was mixed with tinder and formed into small cones which could be burned either directly on the skin or upon layers of soybean paste or small slices of ginger root. Pellets of moxa are now often squeezed on the handle of acupuncture needles and ignited. Moxa is also sold formed into sticks (cigars) which are ignited and held over the spots to be healed. This type of counter-irritation formed of itself a specialty of treatment which served to give a greater stimulus to acupuncture treatments at a time when electricity was not yet available. Many persons with burn scars at acupuncture points testify to the ongoing popularity of this method of treatment in the Orient. Moxibustion is simply another way of applying heat to the body.

Fluid Puncture

This combines acupuncture with the injection of minute amounts of medication at acupuncture points. Local anesthetics, vitamins and hormones are often used in very minute quantities.

Incision and "Prick Open" Therapies

With a heavy needle the skin is pricked open over acupuncture points and the pricking is continued into the subcutaneous fibers. There should be no bleeding and the wound treated with iodine and covered with a dressing. Incisions, 0.5 to 2 cms. long are sometimes made in the skin over the acupuncture point. Subcutaneous, fatty tissue is removed with a hemostat and the blade of the needle is pushed into the opening until a feeling of "teh chi" is experienced.

Suture Implantation

A piece of catgut on a round cutting needle is inserted about 1 cm. from the acupuncture point and is pulled through the subcutaneous tissue in an arc pattern, emerging about 1 cm. on the other side of the point. Ends of the catgut are cut close to the skin and a dressing is applied. This is left in place until eventually the suture is absorbed. The therapeutic effect is presumed to occur from the continuing irritation of the foreign body.

Staples

Although stainless steel staples have been commonly used at acupuncture points, these may cause infection and keloid formation. Such staples are difficult to remove without a special staple remover and, hence, patients have developed infection as well as experienced difficulty and pain in the removal of a staple. The practice of stapling is, fortunately, on the wane.

Scalp Needling

A recent method of needling was developed for the treatment of diseases of the nervous system, particularly such conditions as cerebral hemorrhage, cerebral thrombosis, Parkinson's Disease, chorea, headache and similar afflictions (9). Its basis was felt to be a reflex stimulation of the micro-circulation of the brain from needles placed in the scalp in accord with the localization of cerebro-cortical function upon the projected areas of the scalp. The needles are placed in reference to the underlying brain areas responsible for the type of function to be influenced. Particular attention was thus given to motor and sensory areas topographically located. Language areas, areas of vestibular function, areas of visceral control, etc., are similarly stimulated.

Several needles of 26-28 gauge are placed on the side contralateral to the body region to be treated. The scalp is swabbed with iodine and 2 inch long needles are inserted at an angle under the skin. After 3-5 minutes of stimulation, "teh chi" (feeling of heat, numbness, distention, soreness, etc.) has been reported in the corresponding limb or visceral area. Stimulation is given 3-4 times at a sitting with 5-10 minutes of rest intervening.

ACUPUNCTURE ANESTHESIA

In 1958, there was, in the People's Republic of China, considerable emphasis upon combining traditional Chinese medicine with Western medical science in the treatment of disease. The successful relief of post-operative pain controlled by acupuncture needling led to exploration of the use of acupuncture to replace chemical anesthetics during surgical procedures (10). Initial success with stimulation of ho ku (LI-4) for tonsillectomy, tooth extraction and thyroidectomy led to experiments with other points and their use in a wide range of surgical procedures. Acupuncture analgesia was successfully used for many operations, including major surgery of the neck, chest, limbs, abdomen and brain. It has been used in pneumonectomy and open heart surgery. While originally as many as 80 needles were required, now adequate pain control is accomplished with only two or three needles. Points on the ears, fingers, nose, feet and lips are commonly used.

Complete anesthesia is not accomplished, yet in receptive patients, there is sufficient analgesia so that the patient rests comfortably throughout the operation. The use of acupuncture analgesia permits the patient to be awake and cooperative when that is important, as in brain and thyroid surgery. This technique avoids the slow recovery, laryngeal irritation and other untoward side effects of chemoanesthesia. As a result, post-surgical recovery time is shortened and there is early ambulation and good post-surgical control without undue sedation.

Figures vary on the reported use of acupuncture analgesia for surgical procedures in China, but today it is probably used in 30% of all operations. It is necessary that the patient desire this type of analgesia and is of such a disposition as to be calm despite awareness of the pulling and tugging that occurs during the operative procedure. Patients are given some pre-operative guidance and also tested as to an adequate increase of the pain threshold. Where desirable, some pre-operative medication may be given and an anesthetist stands by with backup chemoanalgesia should this become necessary. Needles are placed 20-30 minutes before surgery and electrical stimulation is started at that time and is continued with varying frequencies of stimulation throughout the surgery.

Although a number of surgical procedures have been successfully performed in the U.S. using acupuncture as a sole analgesic agent, it is unlikely that it will become popular in this country. Patients here are accustomed to being "put to sleep" and awakened when "it is all over". Western trained surgeons are accustomed to a completely relaxed patient and do not care for the delay and uncertainty of a surgical procedure that may be interrupted by the change to chemical anesthesia should that be necessary in the middle of an operation.

ACU-PRESSURE

It has long been known that rubbing or pressing on an area of pain can bring about some relief. Severe pinching to produce bruises (bat goo) is a part of Vietnamese folk-medicine. Finger pressure (Shiatsu), ("shi"-finger, "atsu"-pressure)., has long been a recognized means for modifying neural input to relieve pain in Japanese medicine. Many of the points so used correspond to acupuncture points. Some of the most effective points for producing pain and the disabling of an opponent by means of Judo are acupuncture (motor) points where strong pressure is given directly upon an area of sensitive nerve endings. Experiments in China on animals have shown that strong pinching of the Achilles' tendon can raise the pain threshold. Similarly, the ho ku (LI-4) point in humans has been strongly pressed or rubbed with ice to produce analgesia prior to dental extractions.

Massage in Chinese medicine following the basic formulations of energy flow and yin/yang balance is described for acu-pressure therapeutics (11). Thus, points for massage are the acupuncture points along the meridian lines with deep strong massage used to "tonify" or "bring yang" and with light gentle massage to "disperse" or "sedate" and "bring yin".

Although it has been shown that needles placed in acupuncture points with electrical stimulation produce the strongest neural activation, it would seem that pressure or massage on acupuncture (motor) points may well have some beneficial action. A school for acupuncture massage exists in Peking and a thorough exercise of one's acupuncture points can be obtained for a minimal charge at barber shops in the People's Republic of China.

In The People's Republic of China, the massage of eye points is a routine procedure in all schools where classes stop several times a day and all students participate in this method of treatment in order to strengthen vision and to prevent later eye problems (Figure 15). Several workers in the U.S. have reported upon the use of acu-pressure at headache points as a useful technique for the prevention of a developing headache. Pressure at feng-chi (GB-20), tai yang (EM-1) and ho ku (LI-4), in succession for two minutes on each point has proved successful in reducing the intensity of head pain in a number of our patients.

In the U.S., some non-medical acupuncturists have developed techniques for "acu-pressure" to circumvent legal prohibition against the piercing of the skin with needles. The public, having little real conception of the mechanism of acupuncture, often makes little distinction between acu-pressure, acupuncture and electro-acupuncture.

SUMMARY

It is to be expected that a treatment technique that has existed for 4,000 years would have developed many variations. We have here mentioned

The Exercises

Exercise 1. Close eyes, put thumbs on the *jingming* points, squeeze and press toward the bridge of the nose (8 counts, 4 times).

Exercise 2. Press *taiyang* points with thumbs and with the side of the second section of index fingers massage the upper and lower parts of the sockets, first the upper part and then the lower part (4 counts). Then massage the *taiyang* points with thumbs (4 counts). (Altogether 8 counts, 4 times).

Exercise 3. Massage the *sibai* points at the middle of the lower part of the sockets with index fingers (8 counts, 4 times).

Exercise 4. With index and middle fingers massage the *fengchi* points (8 counts, 4 times).

Exercise 5. Bring fingers together, place them on the sides of the nose, move up to the forehead, pass through the *taiyang* points on both sides and come down (8 counts, 4 times).

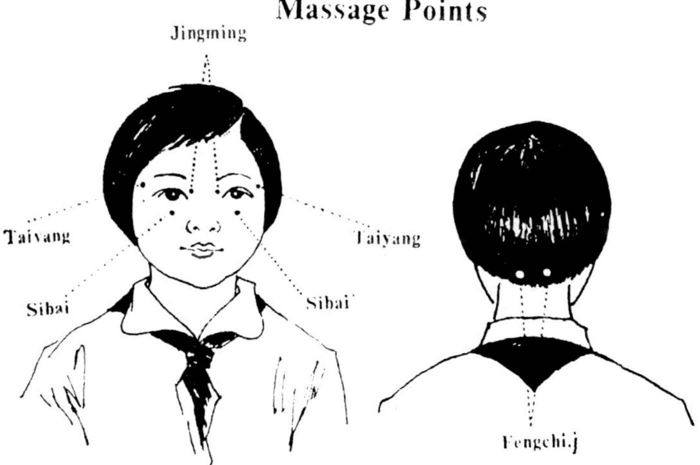

Figure 15. Chinese "eye exam" chart illustrating acupuncture points used for daily massage for ophthalmic hygiene.

only a few. The greatest change of all has been the addition of electrical stimulation combined with the new knowledge of the anatomy and physiology of acupuncture points. With the rapid expansion of knowledge regarding pain mechanisms and pain management, the acupuncture of the future may be as different from that of the present as physiologic acupuncture is from the traditional practices of 4,000 years ago.

C. BRIDGING THE GAP FROM TRADITIONAL TO PHYSIOLOGIC ACUPUNCTURE

"Chinese medicine and pharmacology are a great treasure house and efforts should be made to explore them and raise them to a higher level."*

"No yin, no yang?" Some have already complained that our approach to a modern method of needling based upon physiological facts and theories is not acupuncture because we have left out mention of the balancing of body energies, yin and yang. Our reply is that we are living in the 20th century. It is no longer necessary to hypothecate mysterious forces traveling through non-existent channels. This in no way detracts from the observations of early Chinese physicians. Rather, we must marvel at the precision of their observations and findings at a time when there was practically no knowledge of anatomy or physiology and the everyday tools for diagnosis were non-existent. That there is pertinence for us today in their observations is understandable in that the physiology and psychology of man and the diseases to which he is subject have remained relatively unchanged throughout the centuries. A description of how some theoretical explanations by ancient Chinese physicians anticipated modern scientific thought is fascinating. However, it is no substitute for the use of modern scientific knowledge as a basis for a sound theoretical framework that can be used to formulate and develop a rational therapeutic plan for the most effective placement and stimulation of needles in the treatment of disease.

As we have seen, fundamental to traditional Chinese medical treatment is a concept of energy of life force (chi, chhi, qui). The Chinese were aware of the circulation of the blood long before it was discovered by Harvey, but they had no knowledge of the central nervous system. As it was felt that the life force must take some other pathway it was understandable for them to develop the concept of meridians (ching-lo) as an

*Chairman Mao Tse-Tung, 1953.

acceptable theoretical concept of conduits for the transmission of energy throughout the body.

The concept of yin/yang balance is basic to Chinese medicine. It would not have been unusual for observant physicians, even 4,000 years ago to note the homeostatic balances of the body including such observations as: that the pulse can beat rapidly or slowly, that respiration can speed up or slow down and that blood pressure can raise or lower. The interpretation made would naturally be in terms of the then existing philosophy and the all pervasive balance of yin and yang. Five element theory (fire, metal, wood, water and earth), had its parallel in Western medicine as similar elements were hypothesized by the early Greeks and Romans as basic building blocks for natural functions. The interrelationship of these elements (or functions) was hypothesized as representing the interrelationship of various body organs. This has its parallel in modern medicine where we regularly observe how various organ systems interact in such fashion that the dysfunction of one, for example, liver or lungs can interfere with the function of another, namely the heart or circulation. The elaborate rules of Chinese acupuncture for balancing or remedying such organ interaction dysfunctions in terms of altering the basic five elements is quite logically founded upon multitudes of observations and their interpretation in terms of ancient philosophical concepts. The pervasive utilization of numerology in acupuncture theory is again a function of the beliefs that existed at the time that the practice of acupuncture was developed.

Pulse diagnosis requires a different explanation. Some say that it had its origin due to the fact that, at the time of the development of traditional Chinese medicine, male physicians were forbidden to examine the female body and hence they had to make their diagnoses entirely from examining an arm that was thrust out to them from behind a heavy tapestry. One can picture an ancient Chinese physician convincing himself of the prime importance of facts learned from palpation of the pulse while at the same time, like a physician of today, availing himself of every other bit of diagnostic information that he could gather. Thus, he was surely very much aware of sounds and odors coming from behind the curtain and particularly of the condition of the hand he was examining. In this latter regard it is of note that a recent publication has listed some 70 or 80 diseases that can be diagnosed from simple observation of the hand (12). This art of hand diagnosis has been lost in recent years due to the advent of sophisticated laboratory and diagnostic equipment. But not so to the ancient Chinese physician who, putting it all together, formulated the patient's treatment in his mind all the while carefully palpating the 12 pulses, and estimating some 28 varieties in each of them and attributing all his diagnostic prowess to this sphgmological feat.

One of the most fascinating of these early Chinese observations was that various bodily functions have peaks at different hours of the day and night. Thus, for example, the treatment of lung disease was best done at 4 a.m. and it was said that one should observe the pulse, only in the early morning hours when much of the body was at peace. Such observations presaged the current interest in circadian rhythms of body hormone secretion which forms the basis of the new science of chronobiology which is in an embryonic stage of development.

One could go on for great length in finding similies and grains of predictive anticipatory knowledge in the vast literature of traditional Chinese medicine. Be that as it may, we can only now, as at the beginning of this section, agree with Chairman Mao that indeed ancient Chinese medicine does contain ideas that are pertinent for modern medicine. The renaissance of acupuncture has brought about increased efforts in the area of pain research. New knowledge has evolved and we stand now on the threshold of the development of a scientific and more rational method for the treatment and control of pain.

REFERENCES TO APPENDIX

1. **Veith, I.:** The Yellow Emporer's Classic of Internal Medicine. Univ. Ca. Press, Berkeley, CA., pp. 260, 1949.
2. Porkert, M.: *The Theoretical Foundations of Chinese Medicine; Systems of Correspondence.* MIT Press, Cambridge, Mass., p. 368, 1974.
3. Wu-Wei-Ping: *Chinese Acupuncture.* Translated by Phillip M. Chancellor, Health Science Press, Rustington, Sussex, England, 1959.
4. Needham, J., and Lu, Gwei-Djen: *Celestial Lancets,* Cambridge University Press, Cambridge, Mass., p. 427, 1980.
5. Nogier, P. F.M.: *Treatise of Auriculotherapy.* Maisonneuve, France, p. 321, 1972.
6. Wen, H.L., and Cheung, S.Y.C.: Treatment of drug addiction by acupuncture and electrical stimulation. *Asian, J. Med.,* 9:138-141, 1973.
7. Patterson, M.: (As quoted by Potterton, D.A.) *Ten-Day Cure for Addiction. Bestways,* 9(3):104-105, 1981.
8. *A Barefoot Doctor's Manual.* The translation of the Official Chinese Paramedical Manual, Running Press, Philadelphia, p. 942, 1977.
9. *Yau, P.S.: Scalp Needling Therapy.* Medical Health Publishing Co., Hong Kong, 1975.
10. *Acupuncture Anesthesia.* Foreign Languages Press, Peking, 1972, People's Republic of China.
11. Borsarello, J.: *Massages in Chinese Medicine.* Maisonneure, France, pp. 267, 1973.
12. Berry, T.J.: *The Hand as a Mirror of Systemic Disease.* F.A. Davis Co., Philadelphia, 1963, p. 215.

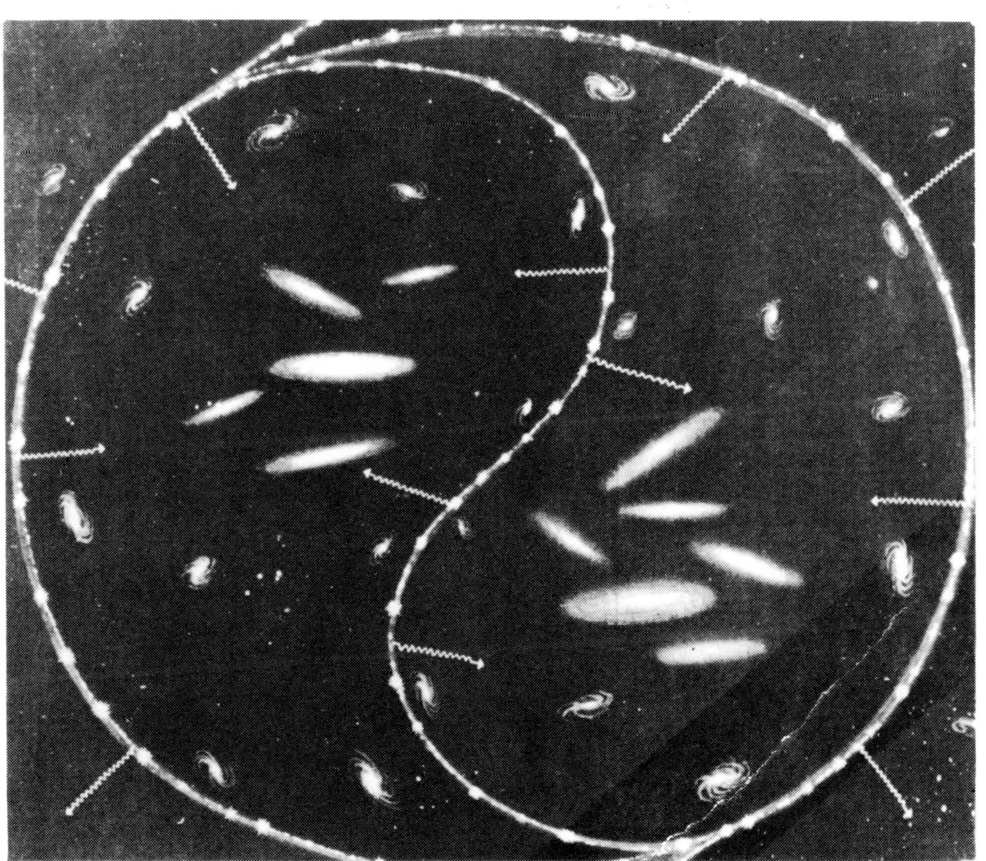

Figure 16. "Theoretical symmetry of Matter and Anti-matter in the Universe" as postulated by Dr. Floyd W. Stecker of the laboratory of Space Physics of NASA's Goddard Space Flight Center. Post Dispatch, St. Louis, Mo., July 31, 1973.

INDEX